SOUND DIAGNOSIS
A HARMONIZED APPROACH TO MEDICINE

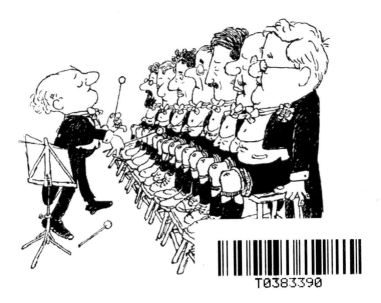

T0383390

MARIA RIBEIRO

with

Gerard Hoffnung's illustrations

Radcliffe Publishing
Oxford • New York

Radcliffe Publishing Ltd
18 Marcham Road
Abingdon
Oxon OX14 1AA
United Kingdom

www.radcliffe-oxford.com
Electronic catalogue and worldwide online ordering facility.

British Library Cataloguing in Publication Data

A catalogue record for this book is available from the British
Library.

ISBN-13: 978 1 84619 208 1

Printed and bound in the United Kingdom by
Hobbs the Printers Ltd, Totton, Hampshire, SO40 3WX

CONTENTS

Dedicated to the Doctors of tomorrow

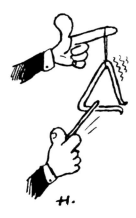

Seeking Sound Diagnostic Direction

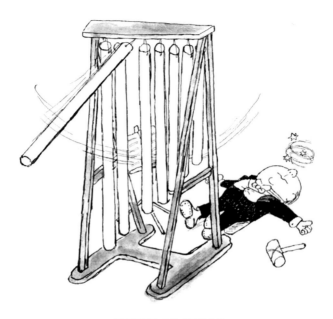

TUBULAR BELLS

Medicine is so very humbling. Stay on the key note. A striking sign or subtle prompting must ring a bell to arouse or awaken our curiosity. Each sounds its own message and beckons until we respond to its real call. If you find a definite sign check its etiology.

APPROACH TO COMMON SIGNS

About the author and illustrator

Maria Ribeiro b.1954, in Durban, South Africa.
Maria specialized in Internal Medicine, followed by a sub-specialty in Medical Oncology. She works as a consultant physician at Kalafong Hospital and the University of Pretoria where she trains senior medical students in Clinical Medicine.

Sound Diagnosis is illustrated by Gerard Hoffnung's endearing cartoons in which the author discovered remarkable connections between the conductor trying to master instruments of the orchestra and the numerous observations that a doctor needs to make in order to reach a sound diagnosis.

Gerard Hoffnung b.1925, in Berlin, Germany.
Gerard arrived in London in 1939 as a schoolboy refugee. From an early age, his gift of observation found natural expression in capturing the elements of music inherent to life.
Gerard died of a cerebral haemorrhage in 1959. He leaves a sweet legacy, a small taste of which you can find in this book.

Acknowledgements

I came upon the art-work of Gerard Hoffnung in 2002 while browsing in the bookshop of the Royal Festival Hall in London. I am delighted to combine the strengths of artist and physician to appreciate the music in medicine and to help you hear the 'symphony' when a problem comes to resolution. (It sounds like …) Suddenly it all comes together to crescendo, just before the diagnosis is made, into a naturally harmonized conclusion.

I would like to record here my sincere thanks to Annetta Hoffnung, Gerard's widow, for granting me permission to use many of her husband's timeless drawings to enhance my work, and for being so instrumental in the whole project.

I thank my mother for lifelong encouragement, and my dear husband and children for their forbearance during the writing of this book.

I am deeply grateful to all students, patients and colleagues who have helped me clarify diagnosis first-hand. Dr. Jurgen Dinkel and Professor James Ker of the University of Pretoria have given very generously of their time and advice toward helping me consolidate pathology in medicine.

I am thankful for each person's valued contribution, from the book's inception - Dr Hannah Brand, Gerard B, Doris, Peggy - through to final design - Vera Brice - and Radcliffe publication.

Maria Mendes Ribeiro
August 2007

KEY SIGNATURE

Employ the systematic approach to clarify diagnosis!

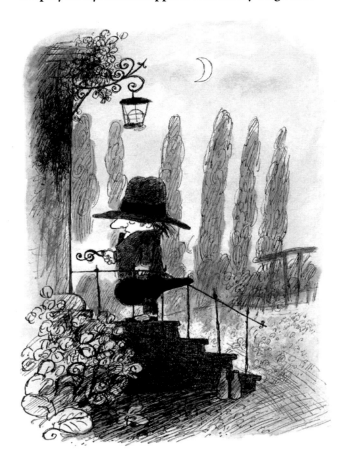

1 AN OVERVIEW OF WHAT LIES AHEAD

Constructing a sound diagnosis

As good practitioners of medicine,
we facilitate the process of diagnosis
by respecting its systematic flow.

Be patient. Listen and be aware.

Conduct your diagnosis with flair –
in three flowing systematic movements:

➤ the 1st is **OBSERVATION**

➤ the 2nd is **EXPLORATION** and

➤ the 3rd is **INTEGRATION**.

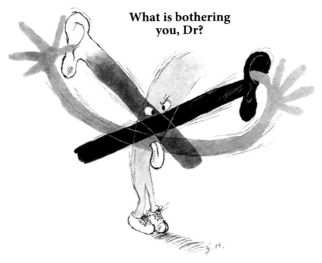

What is bothering you, Dr?

A DISCORD

A baffling case…an unresolved clinical picture …
nothing certain to affirm the diagnosis … I'm trying to orientate
myself … what exactly am I seeing, feeling, hearing?

I would like a **strong lead** to show me the way.

When you want diagnostic support - pause, and get a second
opinion from yourself. The best medicine for a doctor in
distress is to **relax** and **observe the patient**.

Be receptive to the most prominent findings of the often
unexpected pathology that is staring you in the face.

- Attune yourself to what your patient is telling you.

- Align yourself with what you observe.

- **These clinical supporters** are your **strongest leads.**

The body has its own harmony;
We notice this most sharply when any part
plays out of tune.

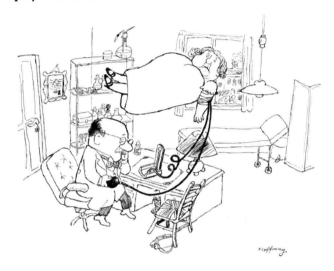

- To identify the cause of the patient's masked presentation, tap into core knowledge - for this resource never runs dry.

- Infuse a clinical picture with increased diagnostic certainty. Only use reliable evidence.

- **Start on a clear note** - with the most striking finding that draws you into the diagnostic problem. The main signs lead the way until they reach a chordant place.

- Try to be systematic to facilitate the 'distilling' process.

OBSERVATION

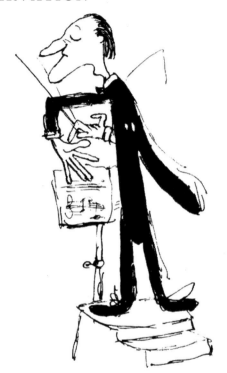

PRECISO

State the main problem
Clear statement of theme.

The sound physician plays it safe.

Our sweet sound of commitment must not fade ... off note.
Stay with your initial observations and concerns.

OBSERVATION

1st movement opens the case.

➤ Your points of reference in diagnosis are the physical signs which your patient displays.

➤ The surest and only way of recognizing the signs is through careful and trained observation.

➤ The careful diagnostician will take steps to confirm and verify the accuracy of the first observations.

➤ Once the leading signs are found, the diagnostician needs the discipline to stay with those signs until their etiology is discovered.

➤ Only through careful observation can an accurate description and all-inclusive differential diagnosis be made.

Main theme is announced

Maestro lets the key notes play and come into view.

Free from assumptions, s/he is OPEN to whatever condition presents itself. Observing the 'major' and 'minor' key signs opens up the main and secondary themes out of which the diagnosis will develop.

What strikes you in your patient?
Notice what you have observed.
Have the confidence to trust your observations.

EXPLORATION

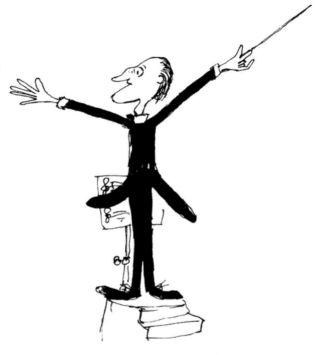

INTRODUZIONE

Focus on the main problem
Follow through the stated theme.
Basics in place, you can now proceed confidently.

EXPLORATION

2nd movement explores the diff diagnosis.

➤ Constantly refer back to basics - they will take you far.
In the 2nd part of the diagnostic process we consider all
possible diagnoses. This is the point where a diagnosis is
most likely to go awry.

➤ Keep it simple. Define the main problem.

➤ To secure different etiologies for that key sign - follow it
through. (Continuity sustains harmony).

Focus on your clearest sign and explore it fully
to widen your perspective to all diagnostic possibilities.
Too many sub-themes confuse and blur the picture.

➤ At each striking sign go back to the crux - i.e. the rich source
of basic pathophysiology to review possible causes from
which a disease entity might stem. Having reviewed these
fundamental mechanisms allows you to move forward
objectively on a sound and broad differential diagnostic
footing.

➤ Developing this sound technique harmonizes our approach
and clarifies our diagnostic route. Our clearest sign and our
core knowledge work together to pull the diagnosis into a
harmonious whole.

**This quick pathological review at the bedside opens
one's vision and field of awareness.**
Harmony, melody, rhythm … i.e. basics of good music.

INTEGRATION

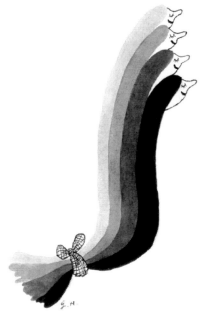

A CHORD

That initial striking feature gains more prominence, and coalesces into a naturally harmonized diagnosis.

Examine the patient 1st.
Define the main problem.
Focus on the problem.
Pause and reflect.
Stand back and reconsider your diff diagnosis.
Keep an open mind.
Let come up what comes.

INTEGRATION

3rd movement consolidates the diagnosis.

> ➤ Having followed the above steps, you arrive at a point from which you are able to take a broad view of the diagnostic panorama.

> ➤ Having viewed the full spectrum and identified some prominent features which have caught your attention, look for other features which you might want to include or (as importantly) exclude from your diagnosis.

> ➤ Having decided what features to include, and which to exclude from your diagnosis, the picture becomes clearer and stronger. Sound diagnosis presents itself and does not need to be forced: suddenly 'it is there' for you.

Maestro, the eminent musicologist of medicine, narrows it down to this one disease process. Weighing up various factors that confront him, he prunes out irrelevant ones that obscure his view, allowing him to focus on the main pathology to verify its presence. He comes to his conclusion - at the end.

The more one can observe - the more one sees - and the more complete the diagnostic picture.

Recapitulation of the main theme
'Putting it all together'

2 A GUIDED CASE PRESENTATION

It is good to see a challenging case. As upcoming physician you will need to be prepared for every eventuality in the unique and complex presentation of patients. In everyday practice we see all colours and variations of the diagnostic rainbow - subtle hues and multi-varied shades of grey. Observe through the discerning eye of the physician for diseases manifest themselves differently.

Many a time signs are not typical or 'text-book' and one may be faced with a diagnostic dilemma. The question is thus: How does one get beyond the inherent uncertainty and ambiguity of presenting symptoms and signs of clinical medicine?

The picture remains undefined until we conduct a full evaluation and appropriate investigations to lay bare the underlying evidence that is available to us.

In Medicine, as in life, there are few absolutes.

Every 'classical' case of Diagnosis

Once decided that the aim is to be
Diagnostician who uncovers what is real pathology
Using reliable diagnostic method turns confusion into clarity
Exposes the 'hidden' malady to yield a targeted remedy

Approaching by means of a confident strategy
Extracts relevant information systematically
First listening, we examine, laying our hands on the sick
For we're only ready when clear features are picked

To elicit and analyse are diagnostic skills that we need
To put into practice all the theory we read
Mastering key signs becomes our guiding melody
Achieving to restore order where there is disharmony

Conduct a case presentation so that it flows

♦ **Get into the rhythm of systematic observation.**
♦ **The diagnosis is already there.** Be open.
♦ **Relax.** You will get there calmly and systematically.

Diagnostic movements
➤ *1st, observe.*
➤ *Next, stop to explore the possibilities.* Practising this discipline allows hidden probabilities to surface.
➤ *The 3rd formulates* into its logical conclusion.

▪ **Dia-gnosis** is made up of two Greek words: Dia is 'looking through' and gnosis is 'knowledge'.
▪ Often a confounding picture: multi-potential etiologies, co-existing pathology, known and unknown contributing factors, compounding complications.
▪ Each patient presents his or her own clinical problem.
▪ To see **unbiased** through the haziness, choose the most conductive pathway to diagnose. A systematic approach provides the framework upon which a diagnosis will unfold, and helps propel the process towards its final goal.
▪ As we elicit clear and pertinent findings, the fog is gradually lifted to reveal an emerging pathology.
▪ Again our systematic approach has contributed in varying degrees toward concluding our diagnosis.

Why does an orchestra need a conductor?

There would be chaos without one. He co-ordinates all the different parts and gives the music shape and body. Similarly, the process of diagnosis puts together the different pieces that harmonize into a presentable whole.

Our **1st movement** is to observe fully.

Set into motion a sound diagnostic journey...

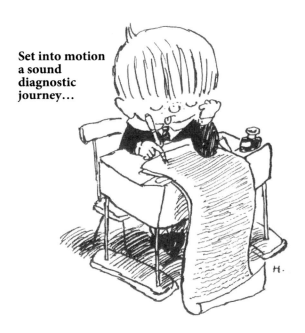

Become sensitized to sights and sounds of disease.

- **Engage all senses** to appreciate and gather valuable information from the very first interaction with your patient. **We want a reliable history and physical examination** to pick up signs that fit together into one complete picture.

CAREFUL LISTENING...
MORE CAREFUL LISTENING

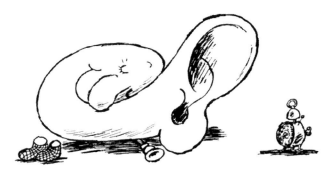

Communicate with compassion at all times!

'Greetings, Why did you come to hospital?'
'My problem ... I feel dizzy ... if I eat I vomit...'
*'Tell me **more** about your problem please.'*

As a prelude ...

➤ **History** 'background' places a problem in context. An **open question** elicits an **open** response that facilitates or accelerates our journey.

➤ Patients express concern related to their *current* condition.

➤ **Listen** without prejudice, intent on understanding.

➤ **Past history** is obtained to ensure that nothing of significance or relevance is missed.

➤ *Pertinent* questions consider possible etiologies and narrow down the pathologies to specific systems. Be alert to pick up on any clues that might be of value.

History-taking illuminates a diff diagnosis.

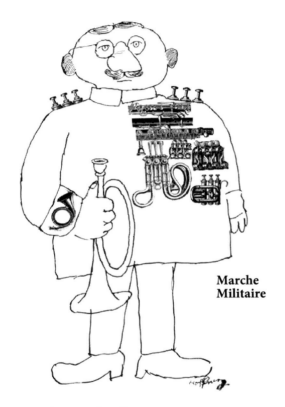

Marche
Militaire

The general examination
Always start with the **general overview.**

As the bugler sounds the advance warning call, so the patient's overall appearance communicates his or her **general condition,** e.g. he or she looks acutely/ chronically ill.

Vital signs

1 Temperature
2 Blood pressure
3 Pulse
4 Respiration

Is the patient …?
hyperthermic - **hypo**thermic
hypertensive - **hypo**tensive
tachycardic - **brady**cardic
tachypnoeic- **brady**pnoeic

Vitals are vital

To indicate cardio-respiratory compromise v. homeostasis and acute v. chronic illness.

These signs are of paramount importance for they signal volumes and tempos out of normal range.

SAFE observations

O_2 saturation
Urine dipstix
Blood glucose!

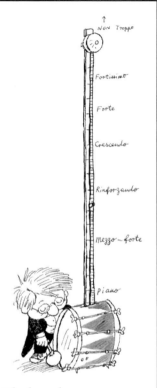

The bass drum

The vitals are so basic

A vital experience - the T°, BP, Pulse and Resp. Rate are being monitored.

The systems examination

At all systems we 1st look, then feel, tap, and listen.

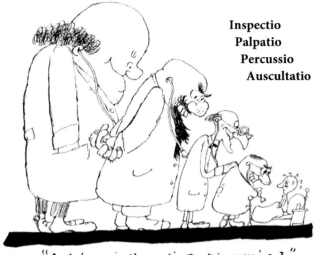

Inspectio
Palpatio
Percussio
Auscultatio

"And how is the patient this morning?"

Keep to the systematic rhythm of observation.

We use the classical Internist approach to *elicit and describe the signs as accurately as possible* to deliver information which brings us closer to the differential diagnosis.

- A quick precautionary check through the systems helps to identify those requiring focused attention.
- Thomas Aquinas said: Nothing except through the senses.
- **Use your senses** to unlock the positive and negative signs that are key to researching and reaching a diagnosis.
- **'We found the problem. We used our senses.'**

OPEN YOUR SENSES and USE THEM ALL.

JACCOL
Jaundice, Anemia, Cyanosis, Clubbing, Oedema, Lymphnodes

In India they say **PICKLE** - Pallor, Icterus, Cyanosis, Koilonychia, Lymphadenopathy, Edema

We can all miss or skip important notes in the score.
Return to check the parts we tend to forget - the eyes, mouth, neck, lymph drainage areas, hands and peripheries.

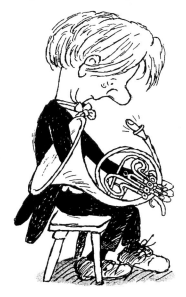

Did you complete your **GENERAL EXAMINATION?**

GENERAL APPEARANCE + VITALS + JACCOL

1st movement over!

Our **2nd movement** is to explore fully.

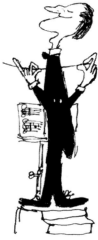

ALERTO

Be alert to common pitfalls that interfere with the peaceful unfolding of diagnosis **as** these may result in an incomplete differential diagnosis and missed pathology.

- No matter the circumstances - be unfailingly systematic!

- Did you fully complete examining the systems in question? Re-inspect incomplete history. Re-inspect examination. Go back to the patient, your primary source of information. **Observation** is **active**. Check the gaps. **Initial accurate** observation excludes most possibilities, directing you to a manageable few. Being prudent motivates us to perform a **complete** and **explorative examination** so that 'seemingly hidden' signs are not missed. Describe your findings.

Have we defined the main problem?

We want the clearest and most unambiguous starting point.

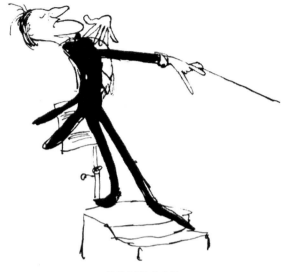

POMPOSO

Now that we have *defined the main problem*, we are standing on more solid ground. We **cannot ignore** or overlook relevant pieces of information for these are stepping stones to diagnosis.

- Never turn your back on a compelling symptom nor a worrying sign. Be sensitive to take your cue from patients. Let them indicate the problem that directs to pathology. Laennec, inventor of the stethoscope, stressed 'Listen to your patient, he is **giving you** the diagnosis'. When the patient is too sick to speak or to co-operate, let the disease speak for the patient. There is always a lead.

- **Molto Importante!** Appreciate the uniqueness of each case. Do not close and tie up the case before you have opened it.

We know that diseases don't present typically, and that unreliable history is part of practice.

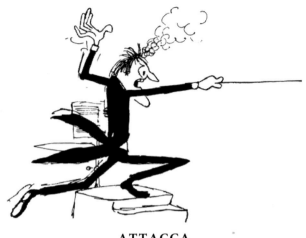

ATTACCA

Do not 'attack' or leap for a diagnosis. Steady on now, Maestro! We do not know the diagnosis yet. It is unwise to jump hastily into a conclusion. A very BIG mistake!

- Do not assume your patient's diagnosis on a single finding before exploring it fully. When we focus too quickly we rush past other possibilities. Avoid letting the history or ambiguous signs direct you too much. Do not ignore, but similarly do not over-react (over diagnose). It is easy to be blindfolded or misdirected by a prominent symptom/sign. To gain a clearer understanding of the patient's pathology, stick with what is certain - those clear-cut signs that you have found or the problem that you have identified, e.g. chest pain: *'So we have identified her problem'*.

- *Do not stray from the main problem that is central to the theme* and thereby prematurely precipitate a Finale.

- We don't have all the information yet. We have to **be patient** for investigations to reveal and unveil the truth.

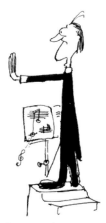

NON TROPPO (NOT SO FAST)

The sound physician waits. 'I want to see a little bit further'. Stop. To become a diagnostician of note, you will need to be more complete in your assessment.

1 *What else did you consider? in your diff diagnosis?*

2 *What are your considerations?*

3 *Broaden your diff diagnosis a little.*

Maintain composure in the search phase for your preparatory examination is done. To see the diagnosis with insight, probe a sign *with insight* for it already knows its way to the disease.

- Expand your view! Delve deeper. Zoom-in on key sign(s). Focus on the root causes of the most prominent sign(s) - those that carry the most weight - and appreciate a quick overview at the bedside. Once you have chosen an inviting direction, stay focused and immerse yourself in your own many-sounded (symphonic) interpretation of the case. This vital movement unlocks acquired knowledge and releases new information as the global picture gradually emerges.

Possible causes? In the 2nd movement we move beyond the most obvious diagnosis of the 1st movement and safely **consider** the **other** possibilities in the whole diff diagnosis.

When weighing up the diagnosis, stay on the key note. Take space and time to assimilate the problem.

What is for *(in favour of)* - **and against** - *each particular condition being considered?* The main clinical lead(s) *in the* **presence or absence** of supporting diagnostic features makes a certain diagnosis **more** (or less) **likely.**

Take into account all relevant and important information in seeking and considering a true diagnosis. **Keep it strong** - only use undeniable evidence to piece together the multifaceted picture. *'As etiology I considered...'*

Be objective and critically appraise your patient. **Keep it open.** If a crucial part of a disease condition is missing, one improvises with a **provisional diff diagnosis** until further evidence reveals the answer. *'I have a diff diagnosis.'*

A discordant note … something that is out of keeping?
When something doesn't fit, look further and openly consider all other diagnostic options. 'Unmatched signs … Not quite fitting … His clinical picture is not quite in keeping… more in keeping with …' This systematic exclusion refines our view.

To appreciate the natural behaviour of a disease, recall its medical name.

'The conductor is there to keep timing, rhythm, and to hear all the instruments harmonize' (Said by a patient).

What is our next step to a good diagnostic workup?

Special Investigations:

1 **Bloods**
   Routines 1st
   Specialized

2 **Imaging**
   CXR
   Appropriate

To reach diagnostic certainty, we use the fountains of wisdom of our colleagues - the radiologist, haematologist, microbiologist, pathologist… Is the **essential information** complete?

$\oplus$ **Proof = hard evidence**

 Initial routine investigations 'cast the net widely'.

- **Blood tests** (haematology and biochemistry profiles) **and X-rays** are **suggestive** of an underlying disease process and may indicate its etiology.

- **More specific tests** point to the diagnosis and unmask the true etiology.

- Ongoing observation & further investigation **provides** sufficient **evidence** to support, confirm, or exclude the working diagnosis. Each clear strand of evidence adds to a greater degree and level of diagnostic confidence.

- If you expose your patient to an invasive diagnostic procedure, ensure it is necessary. Naming the right disease clinches the diagnosis, allowing us to prescribe with therapeutic confidence and deliver service of a high standard.

- Patient is on the mend … Monitor response to Rx. Adjust prescription accordingly. Write instructions legibly so that no ambiguity arises for other healthcare workers. All the necessary has been taken care of. An interlude allows initial individualized treatment to take effect whilst awaiting outstanding results …

…. and then the diagnosis came to light.

Our **3rd movement** integrates all findings

Reflection time - (still a little foggy).
So what have we got here? What strikes you?

- **Stand Back** to ponder the case as a whole and see the diagnostic picture fall into place. Review all information to form your best clinical opinion.

  This pause to reflect allows all facts to settle and the most likely diagnosis to emerge. *'The real sound can be heard: it sounds like, it looks like …'*

- **Gather your impressions** from the **history**, the **physical examination** and the **special investigations.**

The clinical, radiological and blood picture must concur.

Are all in keeping? When something is harmonious, the notes are not discordant. They don't clash!

At this stage- we can appreciate that our systematic combination is the keynote to a sound diagnosis.

Dr, did you follow the steps to diagnostic clarification?

What is your clinical impression? Summarize the problem.
Take out the gist of it which links the past, the present, and the future into a clear line of thought.

NB!

Take a few **extra** minutes to wrap up the case!
Before presenting to your examiners,
'put together' a disciplined summary
in which your **conclusion** comes to the fore.
Structure notes for a more coherent presentation.
Start with a **summary** - without going into the detail.
Next the detail – **In** history, examination, special investigations.

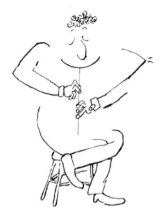

What stands out in your patient?

Define the clinical problem.
Organize and prioritize the case into its true perspective.
Take out the bare essentials - those salient features that bring
together important aspects to form an individual disease profile.

What is the patient's primary problem?

List any 2nd problem/s (probably related).

The picture that comes closest to the most likely cause will
sound like the final diagnosis. There are almost always
unexplained gaps or 'lacunae' in integration.

> You have enough to go on …

NB
Have you prepared a clear case summary?
i.e. ready for presentation?

We want clarity. Once you can write it down, it straightens it
out, to clarify it even further. Now that we have clarified the
picture, keep it strong and succinct. We want a distilled (not
watered down) summary. Don't water down what is good.

In summary:

Present your patient - clearly, simply, systematically.

Patient profile (name, age, gender), ***background***, presenting with
Clinical Problem of: [short and to the point].
Etiology: [Venture a diff diagnosis in order of probability-
        the most likely -
            less likely cause].
Complicated by: [Include all related complications]

Read:

1   **THE SUMMARY *1st*: State final assessment upfront.**
    Introduce a patient with an introductory problem statement
    which sums up the probable diagnosis. The summary must
    include only the major points that are part and parcel of the
    same disease process. A good summary must be **complete**
    and contain all the esssential elements in order to streamline
    your presentation, please your examiners, and augur well for
    success. **Your summary** lights up the background for us. It
    paints a clear and realistic picture of the patient's pathology.
    It must be representative and it must ring true. As more
    information comes to light, the informed summary gets
    shorter and shorter until distilled to its truth.

2   **THE HISTORY: Extract only the noteworthy**.

3   **THE EXAMINATION: Start with the General.**
    Mention only the +ves (notable by their presence) and
    relevant **-ves** (conspicuous by their absence).
    You can demonstrate your findings. **Do not mix** history with
    examination, and **do not repeat yourself.**

4   **THE INVESTIGATIONS: End on a strong note with
    your PLAN: 1 Diagnostic + 2 Therapeutic.**

Does your summary define the problem?
Defining a problem decides the best direction to be taken.
The more summarized the assessment, the more clear-sounding
it will be. Harmony sounds clearly and delights the ear.

The finalist - examiner's corner

Read the notes - it will go more fluidly.
Start with the summary. Don't interrupt the flow. Continue presenting in the same systematic fashion.

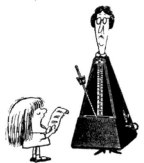

'I am getting a clear picture (of this patient)'

- **Examiner's thoughts:** *Satisfactory exposition.*
  The Candidate is learning to master the signs of medicine.
  It's sounding right. She knows her work. She elicited signs.

- **Physical examination:** *Systematic. Thorough.*

- **Examiner's comment:** *Broadly considered…*
  (or… I don't see enough probity).

- **Common problem:** *'Found signs, but did not explore the causes fully.'*

- **So re-consider and expand your possibilities.** *Diff diagnosis.*

She captured our attention with a case summary that captures the very essence of the problem. It's clarified. She conducts with skill, listening with attention, responding, and allowing the hitherto hidden conditions to surface and reveal themselves. She is precise from the start in naming and describing the signs cardinal to diagnosis. She has disentangled the maze of not so straightforward 'facts' and traced them back to their most probable origin(s).

Suddenly she is face-to-face with the fruit of her labour.

Is your patient-doctor communication clear?

*Quoted verbatim from various patients.

Patient wants to be informed therefore we need to be clear in all our communication.

*I want to know what is wrong with me ...
*and I want to know what is going to happen.

The art of communication is to convey a message that is clear. The only real communication is what the recipient understands.

- **Does your patient (+ family) understand the problem?**

*Relevant and good information is far more helpful to the patient than admonishment. Be truthful in a polite manner.

- Any questions? Address individual needs and expectations.

- Responding to concerns clarifies the patient's condition. As well as allaying fear, it leads to a greater understanding and reassurance of how the problem can be resolved.

- Everything you say and do is important.

- Be precise.

* This doctor is with me, s/he is listening to what I say; s/he is sensitive to how I feel. I appreciate his/her dedication to me.

* I was in need and s/he found out what was wrong with me.

* I feel relieved.

* It is good to be in the hands of a dedicated professsional.

From greeting to parting- we need to be both sensitive and attentive to the way we accompany our patient!

Remember to respect feelings.

*Honouring a patient is part of his or her treatment.

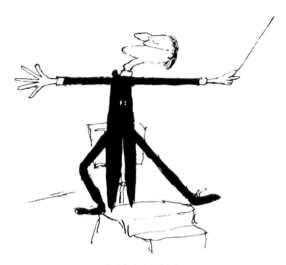

RISOLUTO

Ready to make a sound diagnosis

Always remember the importance of your basics.

Keep firmly anchored to your skills; use them wisely at each level as a safe means to diagnose properly.

Do not neglect them and you will become an observant maestro of medicine.

Go back to basics, so that the concept is there in front of you. Build your diagnosis from a broad and solid foundation. Then you will stand safe and sound with both feet on the ground. Avec de la patience, on arrive à tout.

'The diagnosis flowed to a logical and sound conclusion.'

There is a point in one's career when everything comes *naturally* together and answers come quicker.

Medicus amicus est - **The doctor is a friend.**

'I had the privilege of examining ...'

'(Dr) I appreciate the way you have examined me, and the time spent on me. I will sleep peacefully today.'

'I feel better. Thanks for your time, knowledge and your willingness to help me. I thank you for putting me in the picture so thoroughly.'

I have given my best.

I learn something new from every patient.

The ideal: *A composed manner will inspire your patients' trust, bringing to the consultation heightened awareness, vigilance and sensitivity.*

The real: *The most valuable attention I can accord a patient is my sound diagnostic skill that tries to surpass difficult circumstances ... and my willingness to understand.*

Do what is right for the patient.

'Anyone who is observant and interprets his observations
in a safe and sensible way is a brilliant physician'

Dr Jurgen Dinkel (pathologist)

We lighten our journey when we define the problem and
when we focus on the problem.
Keep fresh - focus on the problem.

Dr to patient: 'You have given me more clarity.'

What do we agree on - the strongest common denominator?
Err on the side of caution with all life-threatening conditions.
Consider and cover all possibilities.

Did you consider any other possibilities in your diff diagnosis?
That unconsidered option must enter one's field of awareness.

- That initial assessment makes a difference. Add value.

- Search with enough probity, look with insight.

We are like Conductors 'through flow'.

Observe - choose your strongest sign - your basics are strong
- follow it through - facilitate the flow of movements in a
clarifying process of diagnosis.

➤ Diagnose from a strong foundation.

➤ Respond to and be guided by leading signs of disease.

➤ Explore your signs fully. Be open to all possibilities.

➤ Analysing is key to gaining more clarity.

A SEXTET

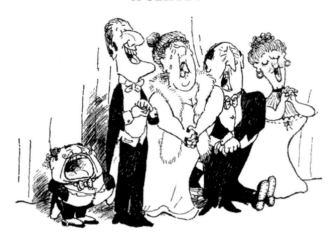

'OPEN YOUR MOUTH FOR ME, PLEASE.'

Be sure to look into your patient's mouth.

'Open up...Ah...Look up.
Does someone have a torch?'

Look at the palate and whole mouth while looking at the tongue.
Simply describe what you see.

3 THE 'BASICOLOGISTS'

Examine
Eyes, mouth, neck, axillae, groins and peripheries for
JACCOL

Your sound entry point to
Basic Signs of Medicine

**Grouped and voiced together in a Sextet to
remember JACCOL**

Here follows a sound approach to **JACCOL.**

Think of all the colours of blood.

[H]yperbilirubinemia / Jaundice

HOW TO RECALL ETIOLOGY?

[A], **B, C, D history**…reviews possible causes
Alcohol - top of the list!
Blood products.
Contacts - viral hepatitis **serology+.**
Drugs - hepatotoxins.
Environment - travel e.g. malaria.
Familial Gilbert's - slight yellowness.
Gallstones - extrahepatic bileduct obstruction - pancreas Ca.
Haemolysis.
Infection viral hepatitis, septicemia, protozoal-malaria.
Immunological hepatitis, cholangitis, cirrhosis.
Infiltration - 1°hepatoma, 2°mets, lymphoma (biopsy).
Ischaemia Hypovolemia - hepatocyte necrosis.

[E]**xamine to elicit signs**
Expose sclerae, mucosae, body to see icterus.
Size of liver? Signs of chronic liver disease:

1 **Estrogenic** = spider nevi, liver palms, gynaecomastia.

2 **Portal H T** = ascites, caput (+ oesophageal varices).

3 **Picture of liver failure** = impairment of functions:

Excretory: ammonia (encephalopathy)? flap - lactulose.
Synthetic: albumin (oedema) + **prothrombin** (bruising).

[M]**andatory** - **liver enzyme** pattern indicates possible etiology:

1 **Haemolytic** [Pre-hepatic] ↑**Unconj B R**, LDH, retics.

2 **Hepatitic** [Hepatic] ↑**Transaminases** ≈ toxic/ infective.

3 **Cholestatic** [Post-hepatic] ↑**ALP** ≈ obstructive picture.

The more severe the obstruction the deeper the jaundice
and the more intense the pruritis. Green skin indicates
predominantly conjugated BR. **Abdomen U/S.**

A, B, C, D history takes you far!

Bleeding / Bruising

Low platelet count / function   or   Low clotting factors?

Examine: Full Blood Count   +   Clotting profile

Etiology: ↓ *production*

Platelets reduced?	Clot prevented?
Thrombocytopenia or Pancytopenia Reticulocyte count ↓ Bone marrow suppression due to:	• **Inherited** deficiency • **Acquired** Synthetic **liver** dysfunction Haematemesis - varices in alcoholic liver failure: Transfuse if Hb low Vit K Fresh Frozen Plasma
1 **infections** - viral 2 **myelotoxin** 3 **infiltration** by TB, malignancy (lympho or myelo-proliferative) 4 **idiopathic aplasia** 5 **vitamin B$_{12}$ deficiency**	**Anticoagulants** **Warfarin** neutralizes vit K dependent clotting factors **Heparin**

↑ *consumption*

Platelets dysfunctional?	Clot dissolved?
1 **Aspirin** (inactivates) 2 **Uremia** 3 **Hypersplenism**-malaria. 4 **Immune-mediated** - ITP, SLE, lymphoma, CLL. Rx steroid + platelet transfusion if bleeding	• **DIC** • **Thrombolytics**

Defect in vessel wall- e.g. trauma, old paper-thin skin, steroids. Severe HT. Telangiectasia - lower lip, bleeder in any part gut.

A bleeding tendency or diathesis- platelet or clotting problem - Exclude a quantitative or qualitative disturbance of platelets or a coagulopathy.

|A|nemia - pale mucosa

|N|utritional? Deficient intake of **Iron, Folate, Vit B**$_{12}$.
A relevant history is N B: Does patient **eat meat?**
Ulcerogenic **drugs, melena stools**. Other visible bleeds.

|E|xcessive blood loss from **G I T**, or non-**G I T** source.

|M|arrow suppression ↓reticulocytes
↓ **R B C production: Causes include:** infective, infiltrative,
idiopathic, myelotoxic, nutritional vit B$_{12}$.
Bone marrow failure = All 3 cell lines depressed.
Bone marrow aspirate (include TB culture), biopsy.

|I|ncreased RBC breakdown ↑reticulocytes = **haemolysis**
Coombs antibody ⊖ : Hereditary RBC defect.
Coombs antibody ⊕ : Acquired immune.
Splenomegaly: Sequestration (pancytopenia).

|A|pproach to anaemia - investigations:

Full Blood Count gives clear direction.
**Include white cell differential count + platelets +
reticulocyte count** (a sensitive indicator of **marrow activity**).

Bone marrow needs the **Haematinics** i.e. Iron, Vit B$_{12}$, Folate.

**'The patient has been investigated high and low -
gastroscope + colonoscope** (stool **occult blood +**)'.

Normal reticulocyte count excludes marrow cause.

HAVE YOU FOUND THE CAUSE FOR THE ANEMIA?

Red cell morphology
Iron deficiency blood picture - red cells small and pale, ↓number, irregularly shaped (aniso/poikilo-cytosis). A **mature person** with Ferritin↓ (?bowel changes) needs to undergo **upper/ lower GIT work-up** to **exclude GI pathology**.
   Appropriate tests e.g. dipstix urine, abdominal sonar.
   Tumour antigen markers, e.g. colon, prostate.

*Bone marrow is the organ of haematopoiesis and therefore requires haematinics and erythropoietin. Check kidney function. Do **iron studies, B₁₂, folate - the full haematinic screen** - on all patients - irrespective of red cell size.*
   We **expect normal-sized** red cells (**MCV**) in **anemia of chronic disease** as well as in **CRF** (due to Fe block in marrow).
Complications of anemia include weakness and heart failure.
   Transfuse a very symptomatic patient carefully.
The **cause** may be **multi-factorial**.
Rx as indicated, e.g. **replace Fe, Vit B₁₂** etc.

IS THE PATIENT A TINGE JAUNDICED?
Anemia with a **recurring lemon tinge** must alert us to possible red blood cell **haemolysis**. ↑Unconj BR, LDH.
Is the RBC haemolysing in the **blood stream** or in the **marrow?**
i.e. Intravascular haemolysis: ↑retics. (Coombs ±).
   v. Intramedullary haemolysis: ↓retics. (↓B₁₂).
Vit B₁₂ deficiency 2° to nutritional or auto-immune pernicious anemia does not allow marrow precursor cells to mature (macrocytes, hypersegmented neutrophils). Sallow skin, smooth tongue, early greying, peripheral neuropathy & mental deterioration (neuron demyelination and axonal degeneration).
   Pernicious anemia is an **auto-immune disease directed against parietal cells** in the stomach. **Antibodies** may be +.
Gastroscopy picture of chronic atrophic gastritis + loss of parietal cells on biopsy. Auto-immune hypothyroid association.
   Reticulocyte response to **i.m. B₁₂** is dramatic.

Know your clubbing members
DID YOU NOTICE BULBOUS FINGERS?

To ascertain whether the patient's fingers are clubbed, view or draw his finger from the lateral aspect. Nail bed hypertrophy becomes apparent. Normally the distal inter-phalangeal diameter measures more than the nail base diameter. When the reverse is true, it is called clubbing.

These patients need a CHEST X-RAY as most causes of clubbing lie in the chest.

Is there evidence of *a suppurative, neoplastic or fibrotic lung condition?* An air-fluid level or lung mass might surprise you.

Can you link *this* basic sign to chronic disease in the:

➤ *Lungs? Pyogenic: Bronchiectasis, empyema, abscess.*
           Paraneoplastic: Bronchus Ca - sick smoker.
           Fibrosis: Chronic hypoxia - velcro creps.

➤ *Heart? Cyanotic congenital HD, IE valve vegetations.*

➤ *Liver? Cirrhoses.*

➤ *Immune-system? HIV, auto-immune rare.*

If no cause is found then it is presumed *familial.*

Is this central cyanosis?

Blue lips, blue **tongue.** *'Patient is strikingly blue'*

Low O₂ saturation of red cells confirmed on ABG.

Usual mechanisms are **acute or chronic hypoxia**.

Elicit signs which **localize pathology:**
- ➤ *In the Heart* - chronic RHF, congenital, mitral valve disease.
- ➤ *In the Lungs* - chronic obstructive or restrictive lung disease.
- ➤ *Between heart and lungs* - pulm. thromboembolic disease.
- ➤ *Outside chest cavity* - obstructive causes e.g. kyphoscoliosis.

Consider a wide differential diagnosis as
many factors can contribute to hypo-oxygenation.

'Heart-lung duet' - cor pulmonale is RV hypertrophy
2° to the above causes, excluding cardiac pathologies.
    The patient's skin is dark, with **plethoric and suffused
conjunctivae** - the **dusky complexion of cor pulmonale** is
imparted to the skin by a **combination of** chronic hypoxia,
hypercarbia and compensatory polycythemia.

Is JVP pulsating - This means a big Tricupid Incompetence.
    He's **hyperinflated** - he has an **epigastic pulsation = RVH**.
    Hear **loud P₂ = pulmonary HT**. **R-heart sounds prominent.**

Investigations show right dominance:

- ♦ **CXR** Big RV + pulmonary arteries = PHT
- ♦ **ECG** R axis. RV strain. P pulmonale - the sign of PHT.
- ♦ **Echo** R side of heart dilated**.**

Said by patient suffering from cor pulmonale 2° to obesity-sleep apnoea:
'The Echo showed nothing that we didn't already know.
    RV enlarged because it's compensating when I struggle to breath.
        The lung function test showed 44% capacity'.
FVC (% predicted).

Oedema?

Best place to elicit is behind medial malleolus.
Possible causes of the swelling? Starling conceptualized **3 forces.**

Elevated hydrostatic pressure
Fluid overload states - Venous congestion due to
severe renal failure, heart failure or constrictive pericarditis.
Postural dependent oedema.

Decreased plasma oncotic pressure
Extravasation of fluid - expect anasarca picture.
All the reasons for a low albumin:
  - ↓ nutritional **intake**, intestinal **absorption,**
  - ↓ liver **synthesis,**
  - ↑ protein loss: **renal** - nephrotic proteinuria.

Excessive permeability of capillaries
a **Infection** e.g. TB pleur**itis**, periton**itis**

b **Inflammation** - polyseros**itis**

c **Malignant** pleural effusion, ascites.

More localized causes
Arterio/veno-occlusive oedema, lymphoedema, cellulitis (warm).
Thyroid - a major organ - pretibial **myxoedema.**

Approach according to pathophysiology
  What is the **mechanism** of oedema?
  Are the **major organs** functioning well?
  You must look at the **heart and kidneys**.
  Has the **urine** been **checked for protein?**
Shall we avail ourselves to **Starling's concept of oedema** to
determine the **cause** for fluid retention?
Rx according to cause e.g. spironolactone.

Oedema comes from the **Greek word O I D E O = I swell**

Lymphadenopathy

Infection
- **Viral**: EBV; HIV as such, + opportunistic-TB, lymphoma, Kaposi. **Epitrochlear LN** a worrisome feature; although suspicious of HIV, may be found in forearm infections, 2° syphilis, lymphoma.
- **Bacterial** local drainage e.g. tonsillitis, STD.
- **Mycobacterial** TB lymphadenitis.
- **Rickettsial** lymphnodes regional to tickbite.
- **Fungal** rare.

Consider uncommon **Immune** or **Infiltrative** cause - sarcoid.

Malignancy - Cervical lymph nodes are a common site for:
- **Solid tumor metastases** from breast, bronchus, thyroid Ca.
- **Lymphoproliferative spectrum:**
  1. **Lymphoma** - arises in **lymphnode**
     - so we expect normal WCC diff.
  2. **Lymphatic leukemia** - arises in **bone marrow** - hence **WCC diff reveals** an **absolute lymphocytosis** in both **CLL and ALL** (>5% primitive blasts if acute).

Analyses
1. **CXR** - looks like? Bilateral **hilar** LN- TB, lymphoma, sarcoid.
2. **Blood tests** might help but **LN biopsy makes the diagnosis.**
3. **Lymphnode aspirate** - MCS, TB culture, cytology.
   (TB lymph nodes may liquefy - caseous pus).

Palpating the lymph node **drainage areas** is part of general examination. Enlarging lymph nodes - an evolving diagnosis? The numerous **big, rounded** and variably sized nodes of **tuberculous or lymphoproliferative disease** are more **noticeable** than a small node which is easy to miss and requires directed and active examination. Narrow the diagnosis down. Check the company it keeps.

Significant lymphadenopathy:
Exclude infection 1st, then malignancy.
'The lymphnode is a world on its own.' *Dr J. Dinkel*

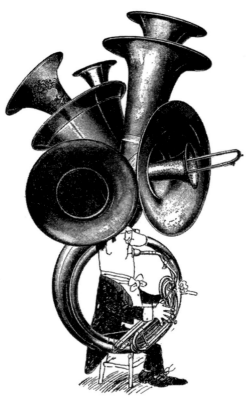

The Great Octuple Bombardon
(Americano Expresso)

THE BASICOLOGIST

So many factors masking the true picture…
We have a system to follow and progress in diagnosis.
Do a good basic workup and assessment for we need the whole systematic combination to make the diagnosis.

4 THE HAEMATOLOGISTS

A recap to get into the rhythm of diagnosis

General examination

Vital signs are vital: temp 38°

Basics J A̲ C C O L̲
Anemia, Lymphadenopathy

Marked mucosal pallor.

- Bone marrow failure - pancytopenia. All 3 cell lines depressed.

- The only evidence of infection in a neutropenic patient might be a high temperature.

- The opposite of anemia - polycythemia - also increases work of the heart. Polycythemia rubra vera - pruritis after bath.

Haematological system

Search for lymphnodes, hepato-splenomegaly.

Fever

High T° arising from? *Let's quickly get to the bottom of this.*

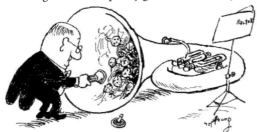

Look for cause *What is the likeliest etiology?*

Infection

Symptoms guide - often vague and misleading, but may point, for example, to a serious lung, renal, heart or bone infection.

O/E Signs direct - run through all systems to find source...

Check resp rate, mouth, ENT, neck stiffness, chest clear? abdo clear? renal angle tenderness, heart murmur ?endocarditis, **urine** dipstix.....a urinary tract infection is a common cause of septicaemia and death, often not suspected in a clinical setting. Rigors (shivers), urine pus cells and leukocytosis strongly suggest pyelonephritis.

- Rickettsial vasculitic rash involves palms + soles.

- T° may be metabolic response to tissue injury.

Pre-antibiotic:

Draw blood and collect urine specimen for **culture.**

Special considerations

- **Portal of entry?** e.g drip site, catheter, fracture **?Staph**

- **Immune compromise?** HIV, DM, steroid, ↓WCC.

- **Anatomical defect?** e.g. prosthetic heart valve.

'Malariologist' says
Always consider and exclude malaria

The most common features of **malaria** are fever, shiverish rigors, ± s**plenomegaly**. The different developmental stages of the parasite (transmitted by an infected female anopheles mosquito) can manifest *in any way* from 'the picture of health' with vague symptoms **plus** a positive travel history - to a very varied multi-system presentation. Do not be complacent - *Plasmodium falciparum* malaria is rapidly fatal if untreated, and can be easily treated with quinine. Preventable †.

Routine bloods may be suggestive of acute/chronic disease, and may ring a bell: F B C helpful - **thrombocytopenia** with malaria, leucopenia in ?Salmonella typhoid - obtunded apathetic patient.
    Confirm infection by + microbial culture or by **direct** microscopic visualization, e.g. + malaria blood smear, or by **indirect** serological antibody detection.

Infective markers are ESR and CRP.

Imaging such as **C X R or U/S** may reveal occult focus e.g. IE.

Malignancy - *Consider non-infective inflammatory response*: *Ca, lymphoma, autoimmune, infiltration when **fever prolonged**.*

Approach - exclude infection. Then malignancy.
Always consider + check for the most common causes of a fever.

Remember to cover the ground
- **Cover** all organ systems
          all possible predisposing risk factors
          all possible infective causes
          life-threatening diseases
- **Consider** the full *microbiological spectrum: Is it: Viral. Bacterial. Mycobacterial. Rickettsial. Protozoal. Fungal. Parasitic?*

Work-up did not yield any specific diagnosis
Fever…'Long time now…even now' and 'I didn't get the
medicine for fever.'   *'The fever bothers me …'*
An unfathomed mystery: Patient is still pyrexial…

Some diseases are occult, and difficult to diagnose.
We need a diff diagnosis. Start with the simple:

➤ **Chronic viremia or TB**, underlying **malignancy.**

➤ **Ca or lymphoma** - a foxy disease, where fever is due to the
   tumour itself, or secondary to bone marrow infiltration and
   failure (neutropenic sepsis).

If they don't fit- then **look beyond the obvious**, to an unusual
'exotic' cause:

➤ **Immunologic** - multi-system **vasculitis**, or

➤ **Inflammatory/allergic** e.g. IBD, or

➤ **Infiltrative '… osis' disease.**

A common cause of a PUO is TB. Granulomatous liver ?TB
picture – a raised ALP and GGT in the presence of a normal
Bilirubin points to granulomatous infiltration by miliary
tuberculosis or sarcoidosis. (biopsy +).

If no diagnosis is reached, be thorough. See case afresh.
Revisit patient with a colleague. Re-examine. Re-assess.
There is always a clue. A urine check, ESR … imaging.

Lymphadenopathy - LN biopsy: therein lies the diagnosis.

'A febrile illness of unknown etiology. Possible osteo - myelitis.
Pyrexia of unknown and uncertain origin - and now is pyrexia of
possible origin, probable origin. T °40
- In the end it was his joints - septic arthritis.'

More often than not, it is difficult to pinpoint a diagnosis, but
once in a while it is spot on e.g. CSF microbiological evidence of
meningitis.

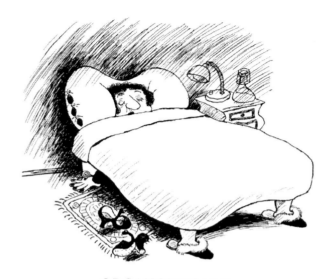

ORGANOMEGALY

Consider an Infiltrative disease. Deposition of iron or amyloid in major organs leads to unusual presentations…
A patient **Lady 'Osis'** developed…

1 **Haemochromatosis - organs commonly infiltrated:**
liver (hepatomegaly - cirrhosis) + pancreas (IDDM) + heart (CCF) + skin (bronzed) + pituitary and gonads (loss of body hair). High serum ferritin; iron overload on liver biopsy.

2 **Amyloidosis** is diagnosed on biopsy (tongue, rectum etc). Renal infiltration presents with nephrotic syndrome.

3 **Sarcoidosis** Skin lesions + hepatosplenomegaly.
Skin biopsy to aid the diagnosis.

Hepatomegaly

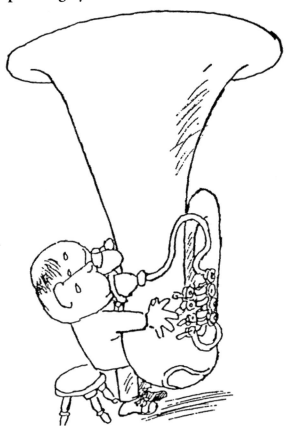

CAUSES: USE CLIMATE

Common causes of tender hepatomegaly are congestion
and malignancy secondary to solid tumour metastases.
Slight enlargement is expected in infectious or toxic hepatitis.

Congestion due to congestive (or rarely constrictive) **HF**

➤ **RHF?** Tender liver, ↑**JVP**, peripheral edema - match up.

➤ Pericardial constriction or tamponade is an often unconsidered form of 'CCF'. 'Heart in armour' restricts filling and emptying. Does the patient have a Kussmaul JVP sign and a weak, rapid pulse?

Liver disease - cirrhosis, fibrosis
Does the patient have an enlarged liver?
　　Always be sure to check upper border; the normal hepar spans 12cm in the mid-clavicular line, from 5th ICS to costal margin, in the non-hyperinflated chest.
Most cirrhotic livers are micronodular and therefore impalpable with the exception of a mixed micro-macronodular cirrhosis associated with chronic Hepatitis B; and haemachromatosis.

Infection - **viral** *hepatitides,* **bacterial, mycobacterial, protozoal** *malaria, amoeboma,* **parasitic** *bilharzia mansoni.*

Infiltration - fatty liver conspicuous on U/S '**... osis'** group.

Malignancy - (hard nodular) ↑ALP + GGT.
1° hepatoma, 2° metastases, lymphoproliferative.

Alcoholic or toxic hepatitis

Tests: CXR, cardiac and abdominal ultrasound.
Before liver biopsy check platelets and clotting profile
- prevent bleed.
LFT. Hepatitis serology. Ca markers - AFP, CEA.

Extramedullary erythropoesis –osteomyelofibrosis.

Splenomegaly

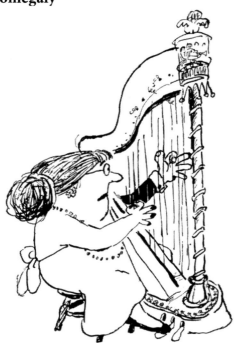

Could this be Gerard Hoffnung lending me a helping hand?

A palpable spleen? Don't 'dig' for an enlarged spleen.
It will tip your fingers when the patient inspires; or turns onto right side. One cannot get in above spleen; percuss for splenic dullness in lower intercostal spaces.

- In most cases, it is not strikingly big - a slight enlargement is common.

- A **massive** firm spleen below the costal margin is obvious in **hepatic schistosomiasis** or in **chronic myeloid leukaemia.**

Congestion due to **portal** HT.

Liver disease - fibrosed liver + congestive splenomegaly
   Liver fibrosis - 2° to hepatic Bilharzia S. mansoni
   Liver cirrhosis - ascites usually conceals spleen.
   Clinical + U/S features of Portal HT?
   Small liver with coarse parenchyma.
   Portal vein dilated with reversed flow direction,
   Congested spleen, Caput collaterals.
   Gastroscopy ?oesophageal varices.
   Pancytopenia 2° to hypersplenism.

Infection - moderately prominent soft spleen:

➤ **viral** - EBV, CMV

➤ **bacterial** - septicaemia - **typhoid**, brucella, SBE.

➤ **mycobacterial** - disseminated **TB**

➤ **protozoal** - **malaria** (tip of spleen), parasitic.

Immunological **I**nfiltration rare 'osis' group

Malignancy: typically haematological etiologies:
Myeloproliferative CML WCC diff (↑granulocytic precursors).
   Lymphoproliferative lymphoma likely if big liver and LN+.
   Solid tumour mets to spleen **unusual.**

Anemia - haemolytic process e.g. haemoglobinpathy.

Tropical endemic malaria spleen big, hard, chronic, immune.

Etiological approach – it's simpler than it looks.

**A few basic causes, similar to those of hepatomegaly,
cover a great deal of ground.**

Hepatosplenomegaly

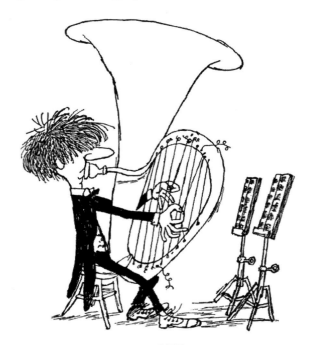

Use **CLIMATE** again.

Reading the causes of a large spleen and large liver

These two organs, in most cases, are not strikingly big - a slight enlargement is common. Both are homogeneous, therefore look alike on sonar. There is an overlap of the same grouping of diseases that cause the liver and the spleen to enlarge, with differences in types of infection. Once on top of basics - diagnoses can proceed. Weigh up everything-consider the most likely causes.

Congestion of both organs may be **2° to severe congestive** (or rarely constrictive) **heart failure or:**

Liver disease with portal hypertension
➤ **Fibrosis - hepatic bilharziasis.**
Early S. mansoni infection enlarges liver slightly; later it becomes firm & nodular, often smaller than normal but doesn't shrink totally as in alcoholic cirrhosis. Bilharzia serology +. Liver / rectum biopsy reveals ova **granuloma** elicited by thousands of eggs laid by female worm in portal circulation. Periportal pipestem fibrosis-U/S image. Liver cells remain normal - preserving their synthetic function; therefore LFT, albumin and prothrombin are normal.
Rx Schistosomicide - praziquantal.

➤ **Cirrhosis** - mostly micronodular; spleen is also usually impalpable. Mixed micro-macronodular picture occasionally**.**

Infection: **viral** - *hepatitis*
bacterial - *typhoid, SBE (congested liver + splenitis)*
mycobacterial - *TB*
protozoal - *malaria*
parasitic - *bilharzia (fibrosed liver - congested spleen)*

Infiltration '... osis' group

Malignancy being RES[1] **organs we expect:**

➤ **lymphoproliferative** - the lymphomas, leukaemias.

➤ **myeloproliferative** - CML - spleen prominent, liver less so.

Anemia - haemolysis.

Tropical disease - malaria.

Extramedullary erythropoesis rare - myelofibrosis
- massive HSM

---

1 Reticulo Endothelial System

Lymph nodes, liver and spleen

This clinical picture presents few diagnostic options.
    The **two main pathologies are TB and lymphoma**.

Infection
TB takes pride of place; infects most organs but has predilection for those of the RES. CXR - Hilar, para-tracheal nodes?

Immunological e.g. lupus.

Infiltration sarcoid - involves same systems as TB - both 'osis'.

Malignancy
Lymphoproliferative lymphoma; chronic lymphatic leukaemia.
The liver is a common site for solid tumour metastases, compared with the spleen, which is more prone to direct invasion by a GIT malignancy.

Approach
Exclude TB and lymphoproliferative malignancy.

| 'Tough bacillus' **Tuberculosis investigation** Lymphnode aspirate Caseous necrosis material TB bacilli+++

 It's TB. It's confirmed. Diagnosis is made. Now we know the name of the disease. | 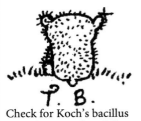
 Check for Koch's bacillus TB culture result to follow |

Just as big lymphoma nodes shrink with lympholytic steroids, big TB nodes 'melt' with TB Rx.

Biopsy of lyphnode gives best yield at end of the day.

Sarcoidosis

An unusual case, **Lady Sarcoid 'osis'**
Multi-organ infiltration, a **granulomatous** disease
'A dermatologist got to the bottom of it -
he took a skin biopsy from my nose.'

Like TB clinically + radiologically + histologically.

Involves eyes + skin + lymph nodes, RES, **lungs ...**

Many a sarcoid patient is mistakenly treated for TB.

Approach to diagnosis?

CXR - suggestive of TB. Hilar LNs ± infiltrates.

- **Sputa** - for TB. ??TB. No proof → look for Sarcoid.

- **Suggestive evidence** - ↑ globulinemia, mild calcemia, ACE.

- **Tissue biopsy is diagnostic** - naked granuloma i.e. inconspicuous inflammatory rim - no caseous necrosis.

Lesions shrink to nothing on steroids.

Treat if sarcoid interferes with major organ functioning, e.g. heart block, lungs - mixed restrictive and obstructive (bullous) disease. Manage iatrogenic Cushing's.

'I was coughing. Doctor thought I had TB.
I had Rx for TB (a long time).
I was at Eye clinic - uveitis - chronic (intraocular inflammation).
Referred to Internal clinic: Sarcoidosis.
I lost weight, I couldn't see...
I couldn't walk. Everything was deteriorating. I was thin.
They put me on steroids. Now I can walk, exercise.'

The disease responds well to steroids.

Large parotids (lift earlobes). Parotis = next to ear.

Infection viral parotitis - mumps, HIV.

Idiopathic **Infiltration** - Sarcoid **Immunologic** - Sjogrens.

Metabolic syndrome

Alcohol most common cause of bilateral parotomegaly
v. unilateral parotomegaly: infection, tumour, lymphoma.

Deep skin pigmentation

Inflammatory - post-inflammatory hyperpigmentation.

Malnutrition - pellagra hyperpigmented sun-exposed skin.

Melanodermia - Addison's (adrenal failure).

Too much iron

O₂↓ Cor pulmonale

Pigment ↓ 1 post-inflammatory - hypopigmentation.
            2 localized - autoimmune vitiligo.
            3 generalized - no melanin in albinism.

Approach to cachexia

Loss of body mass - **weight loss+++**
    To appreciate wasting of fat and muscle expose the chest.

Infection - chronic-viral, mycobacterial 'consumption'.
    Infiltrative or Immunological disease.
    Immobilization.
    Malnutrition Malabsorption.

Malignancy - consider a highly treatable lymphoma.

Metabolic
Diabetes 'is starvation in the midst of plenty' (Ganong).
    Endocrine hyperthyroidism, DM (type1) TSH? glucose?
    Organ failures, e.g. COPD. ↑Work of the failing organ.

Auto-immune

Did you discover the cause?

Have you considered *all* the disease groups?

A good place to start is with nutritional intake.

'My body definitely told me there was something radically wrong. No energy. None whatsoever.'

A wasted patient - ribs prominent - constitutional symptoms - drenching night sweats - the sedimentation is high - CXR picture suggestive of TB.
Do we have a proof of TB yet?
Awaiting sputa onfirmation.

To diagnose TB one needs a high index of suspicion.

Cachexia continued...

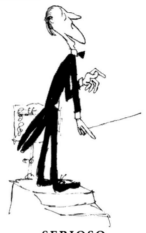

SERIOSO
I'm listening to Mozart's Requiem...**chronic disease.**

Investigations are guided by age and clinical picture.
Keep your options open in considering diff diagnosis.
Emaciated youngster may have a gonadal germ - cell tumour.
TB is a disease of all ages and 'consumes' the patient.
Lymphocytes predominate in tuberculous effusions.

ESR >100 suggests:

➤ **Infection TB** - chronically raised fibrinogen.
➤ **Inflammation** - high se-protein minus low albumin = high globulin fraction. Analysis of hyperglobulinemia by protein electrophoresis differentiates a diffuse **polyclonal** gammopathy from a distinct **monoclonal** band, usually of myeloma. Red cell-rouleaux formation.
➤ **Myeloma** and other **lymphoproliferative** diseases.
➤ **Albuminuria** - nephrotic syndrome.
➤ **Auto-immune disease** e.g. lupus or rare vasculitis.

5 THE RHEUMATOLOGISTS

General examination

Vitals Chart: Temperature?
Basics: Anemia of chronic disease.
Note: hands and nails.

Locomotor examination

'Sore joints' = arthralgia.

'My body and my joints. My whole body is not well.
I became worse…my skin'.

'Tell me about your problem?'
Patient will show you **which painful joints** are involved.
Joint damage + pain limits articular range of movement.

Describe signs observed. Functional impairment.
Is it part of a systemic auto-immune disease?
Are there extra-articular signs?

X-rays are helpful in rheumatology.
Clinical signs may not be obvious.

There are more than 100 types of arthritis.

Here is an easy approach to the arthropathies…

Joint pain   Is this Trauma-related? Or due to:

Osteoarthritis
A degenerative joint disease with an inflammatory component.
Cartilage surfaces in **weight-bearing joints** become irregular.
Later joint unit fuses. **X-Ray** changes (1) osteophytes, (2) joint
space narrowing, and (3) subchondral sclerosis.
1° ageing or 2° to: trauma, sepsis, all **other forms** of arthritis.
Gelling is a common feature; inactivity stiffens the joints
making it difficult to re-initiate movement.
Recovery from stiffness is quick.
Valgus and varus deformities occur in severe cases.
Bony nodules develop at proximal and distal finger joints.

Inflammatory arthritis
a   **Gout** – *monoarthritis:* Rx acute - colchicine, chronic -allopurinol.
b   **Rheumatoid** - *polyarthritis:* methotrexate if active, cortisone.

Infective arthritis
Septic arthritis - Is usually **monoarticular**, and destructive.
A warm hypersensitive joint that cannot move and cannot be
touched! TB arthritis can exhibit similar features but tends to
present with a less sensitive 'colder' joint (like a cold abscess).
Drain surgically.
Reactive arthritis - TB, gonococcus can give sterile effusions.
Polyarthritis may be part of a systemic viremia or bacteremia.
Acute rheumatic fever is a rare possibility.

Neoplastic Paraneoplastic arthropathy in bronchus Ca is rare.
Hypertrophic **P**ulmonary **O**steo **A**rthropathy.

Treatment - rest, analgesic, N S A I D s, specific Rx.

Often the cause of a hot swollen joint is not initially apparent.
Aspirate an effusion → crystals, bacterial and TB culture.
The right way - the classical way - diagnose by aspiration.

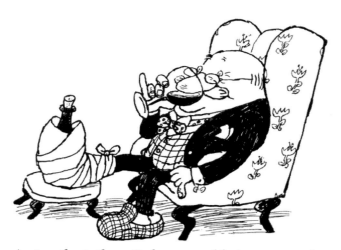

Acute arthropathy ... Podagra ... red foot ... severe pain

Gout is an intense crystal synovitis, intermittent, hereditary.
   Precipitants include diuretics, alcohol, dietary purine excess, or any severe stress such as illness, dehydration, high catabolic state with increased turnover of nucleic acid, and trauma to old gouty joints. Crystalluria predisposes to kidney stone formation. Asymptomatic hyperuricemia is part of a metabolic disease. Primary gout usually involves (one) lower limb joint(s) and can progress to upper limbs and peri-articular soft tissue. In chronic tophaceous gout multiple deposits of pasty gouty tophi are present on hands, feet, elbows and pinnae of the ears.

'I never let them (aspirate) - I couldn't imagine anyone with this severe pain let a physician with a needle anywhere near them.'

COULD THIS BE SLE?

We require 4^+ classification **criteria:** Are there any distinguishing features that may implicate an auto-immune systemic vasculitis?

Polisystem involvement:

Oral ulcers

Skin	Photosensitivity
	Malar butterfly rash
	Discoid lesions
Joints	Polyarthralgia, arthritis
Kidneys	**Renal dysfunction**
	Nephritis - HT, oedema
	Haemato Protein**uria**
Serositis	Pleural/ pericardial rubs
CNS	Most unusual presentations
Blood	↓Hb ↓WCC ↓platelets
	+ANF ... titre high
	Anti-double-stranded DNA

Consequences of immunosuppressive therapy include increased susceptibility to opportunistic infections **and** corticosteroid complications such as peptic ulcer disease and osteoporosis.

Normal CRP helps distinguish this **systemic inflammatory condition** from infection. Nebulous picture - in the end she had an immunological problem - **multi-system involvement - in keeping with SLE** - dermatitis, thrombocytopenia …
Check ANF and ESR.
'Bring it together.'

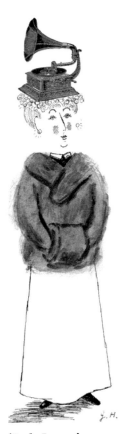

'Lady Lupus'

Immune - mediated diseases affect more Ladies than Lords.

Lupus is always a consideration in an unusual picture.

DOES THE PATIENT HAVE RHEUMATOID ARTHRITIS?

We require at least 4^+ classification **criteria:**

▶ **Articular signs:**
Poly-arthritis ≥3 joints. As a synovitis, **all synovial joints** may be affected. The back is normally uninvolved, excepting for the **upper cervical spine** articular process.
Is it bilateral? The **hands** notably involve the
PIP joints swelling + feeling of bogginess, spindling of fingers + **MCP joints** + **wrists**.
How do patients feel when they awaken in the morning?
Prolonged morning joint stiffness. All joints are stiff + painful. The main diagnostic feature is erosive joint damage.
If we see **cystic erosions** on **hand X-rays** call that disease RA. Classic hand deformities develop. Interossei muscles atrophy.

▶ **Extra-articular involvement:**
▪ **Skin nodules** (extensor forearm surfaces), **eyes.**
▪ **Chest** - pleuropericardial effusion, ILD.
▪ **Blood** - **rheumatoid factor** may become +.

'It took a long time before the doctor gave my disease a name.' Check auto-immune serology.

Diff diagnosis ?   **Auto-immune disease.**
                       SLE alone or a variation.
                       Check criteria.

1 **Overlap syndrome** combines SLE + RA.
2 **Systemic Sclerosis** Scleroderma - diffuse fibrosis – **Raynaud.**
3 **Polymyositis** pain in muscles - proximal muscle weakness.
4 **Mixed connective tissue disease** components of 1, 2, 3.

ANF and RF are part of the picture. Antibodies to Extractable Nuclear Antigens narrow-down diagnosis.

Backache / Bone pain

Orthopaedic causes: Palpation tenderness?

1 **Musculoskeletal** - **d**iscogenic.

2 **Trauma or osteoporosis** - compression fracture.

3 **Infective** - **o**steomyelitis post-spinal surgery.

4 **TB spine** - **o**steitis—collapse > thoracic vertebrae.

Non-orthopaedic causes

Neoplastic: X-ray? wedge-shaped vertebral bodies.
   Spinal cord compression - paraplegia – dexa – RT.

1 **Prostate Ca** sclerotic mets ↑ALP, PSA. Bone scan+.

2 **Breast Ca** lytic mets>sclerotic thus ↑calcium +ALP.

3 **Myeloma** - triad clinches diagnosis:
   a **Lytic lesions** - fractures - **vertebral (2° kyphosis).**↑*calcium*
   b **Monoclonal band** in blood + U-Ig electrophoresis.↑*protein, ESR*
   c **Immature plasma cells** infiltrate >10% bone marrow. *BM failure*

Referred pain:
   Infective - pleuritis, pyelonephritis.
   Ischaemic - MI, aortic dissection.
   Urinary or GIT- e.g. stone, pancreas.
   Neuropathic - e.g. Herpes zoster.
   Paget's - Bisphosphonate for rising ALP.

Enthesitis + spondyloarthropathies

Inflammed tendon insertion sites. Young males. Joint stiffness.

1 **Ankylosing spondylitis - sacroilitis.** X-Ray: Fuzzy S-I joints; inflammation (and calcification) progresses up the vertebral ligament. 'Bamboo spine' restricts chest movement and neck. 'Patient cannot see the rising sun.' HLA-B27+.

2 **Psoriatic arthritis** involves DIP joints (like OA); skin, nails.

3 **Reactive arthritides**. Lower limb joints.

4 **I B D** affects extra-spinal collagen.

CRIPPLING BACKACHE

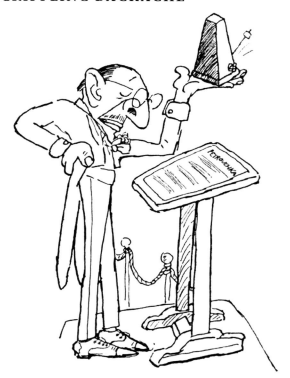

'Pain in back - after a bit of effort it eases.'

It sounds locomotor. Mostly mechanical. X-rays.
The physician must exclude infection and malignancy.
Check blood calcium and ALP to indicate bony lesions.
Leg weakness. Bladder / bowel function intact?
MRI if neurological fallout. Biopsy.

6 THE CARDIOLOGISTS

General examination
To get into the CVS rhythm
A tactile examination suits CVS exploration.

Position patient @ 45° to examine JVP. General condition.
Pause at the pulse. Is it **regular** in volume and rhythm?
Vitals. Check for ↑ J V P $\boxed{\text{JJ}}$ A C C O L $\boxed{\text{TT}}$ Thyroid Trachea

Cardio Vascular Examination

Inspectio:
NECK! JVP, arterial pulsation, thyroid.
Chest wall - **visible**: deformity, op scar, pulsations.

Palpatio:
LV   Localize + characterize **apex beat**. (turn patient on L side).
RV   Left parasternal heave (or epigastric pulsation) = RVH.
Thrill   Palpable murmur - valve stenosis or congenital defect.

Percussio: verifies the limits of heart borders.

Auscultatio: Use the Z approach. Start at apex.
Heart Sounds -Listen to S_1 and S_2 over **all** valve areas-M, T, P, A
and extra pathologic S_3 over L V in L V F, and over R V in RVF.
Murmurs - over each isolated valve - systolic, then diastolic.
Bruits - neck for carotids, abdomen for renal arteries in 2° HT.
Did you check for signs of **heart failure** and **endocarditis**?

Go step-by-step. **Leave the stethoscopes for last!**
Being systematic *will get you to the diagnosis.*

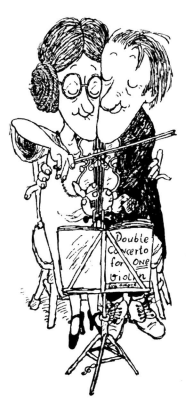

Orchestral hierarchy

The principal violinist is the Head of the Orchestra - the one closest to the conductor.

CORDIS - pertaining to the heart.

2 hearts beat as 1

Feel the L	**Listen to the L**
Feel the R	**Listen to the R**

Causes of Heart Failure

Any disease that involves the heart structure - i.e. peri-cardium, myo-cardium, endo-cardium or the heart's electrical conduction system. On occasion the cause lies outside the heart i.e. extra-cardium.

Observation Symptoms + signs = Stage C Heart Failure.

Roentgen chest signs

Heart large- cardio-thoracic ratio>50% = Cardiomegaly.

   LV hypertrophy - 'sagging breast' configuration.

Picture of LVF: Pulmonary congestion = fluid-filled lungs- 'bat wings', upper lung vessel congestion, interstitial oedema, fluid in fissures (pulmonary venous HT).

   RV hypertrophy - 'proud breast' configuration.

   Prominent conus = Pulmonary artery HT.

   On lateral view RV surface contacts >1/3 of retrosternal area.

Diagnostic bloods, ECG, echo image fit in with ...

Impending complication

Dysrhythmic heart. Systemic (arterio/veno) thromboembolism.

   Poor cardiac output subtly deteriorates renal function, and end-stage hypoperfusion leads to multi-organ insufficiency.

Strategy for antifailure Rx Position upright + O₂

Symptom relief: Diuretic - Furosemide (higher dose needed in cardiomyopathy or in renal impairment).

   Digitalis improves contractility and decreases heart rate.

   Drugs that address the **neuro-hormonal aspect** improve outcome: ACE-inhibitor, beta-blocker, aldosterone-blocker.

   Rx precipitating factor and Rx cause.

The pulses ... a very good place to start.

Are all pulses present and synchronized?
Pulse character may indicate diagnosis.

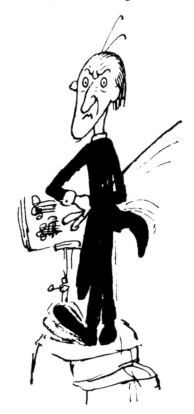

INTERRUZIONE

An irregular pulse! A conductive interruption.

CAUSE AS TO WHY CARDIUM HAS FAILED

*The dominant feature**

1 **Pericardial?** *Pericarditis = Friction rub**
   Infective - viral (e.g. Coxsackie), bacterial, T B.
   Immunological - post-strep rheumatic fever, lupus.
   Ischaemic - Dressler's post-infarction.
   Metabolic - uremic, thyroid disease.

2 **Myocardial?** *Displaced apex + S_3 gallop**
   Degenerative - H T + ischaemic cardiomyopathy is common
   Infective - viral myopericarditis, rheumatic pancarditis !tachy
   Idiopathic - dilated C M O.
   Infiltrative - rare '… osis' group.
   Inherited - congenital heart disease.
   Metabolic - diabetes, thyrocardiac.
   Toxic - alcohol, anthracycline.
   $O_2\downarrow$ - hypoxemia - **Cor pulmonale** - PH T.
   Peri-partum.

3 **Endocardial?** *Valve lesion = murmur**
   Structural : **Degenerative** - AS, MV prolapse.
                     Infective - rheumatic, endocarditis
                     Ischaemic - Chordae rupture.
   Functional : **Myopathic** - dilatation of the heart.

4 **Electrical rhythm disturbance?**

5 **Hyper demanding situations?**

   Additional strain outside heart like anemia, fluid overload,
   lung infection, hyperthyroidism can precipitate patient into
   H F. Hyperkinetic syndrome is really a temporary failure; no
   heart lesion yet heart can be dilated, i.e. precipitants of H F
   in cases of **borderline heart function**.

H F is the end result of a constellation of diseases.

Acute exacerbation of Heart Failure
WHERE IS THE PRECIPITANT?
In Heart? Infarction, atrial fibrillation, valve infection.
    Outside heart? Uncontrolled BP, PTED, etc.
    With patient? Rx Non-compliance.
    With Doctor? Incomplete prescription.

The heart initially copes with increased workload.
Compensatory mechanisms lead to a vicious cycle that causes
the heart to tire and the lungs to weep.

Every cardiac patient gets a diagnostic trilogy:

1 **Chest X-Ray:** to view (size + shape) of heart.

2 **ECG tracing:** to record the electrical activity.
   Scan 'eyeball' ECG for rate, rhythm, axis.
   Every beat is in sinus rhythm-the P-QRS-T wave is complete
   and synchronous with fundamental frequency of SA node.
      How to determine axis: Look at **I** and **AVF.**
   As a rule of thumb: the axis is normal when both are +.
      Left axis I+ AVF - and vice versa for Right axis deviation.
      Small complexes ++fat/ fluid/ air block electrical current.

3 **Ultrasound echo:** to picture heart structures + function.
   Sound waves can bounce back a history.

Stage ABCD classification for heart failure
A Risk factor for heart disease, e.g. HT.
B Structural damage (echographic evidence).
C Symptoms and signs of HF.
D Refractory to medical treatment.

'I have to walk very slowly - take my time and walk.'

Heart failure:
Is the patient in **LHF** or **RHF** or **BVF**?

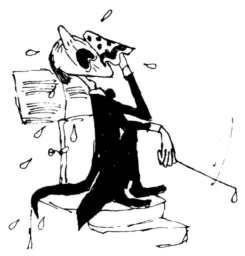

MOLTO DOLOROSO
Pulmonary oedema ~ LEFT ventricular failure

A deeply symptomatic patient… 'I must get O_2.'

Symptoms: Retrograde: dyspnoea, orthopnoea, PND.
Anterograde: poor cardiac output - fatigue,
decreased exercise tolerance.

Signs: (1) Bibasal crepitations, (2) tachycardia,
(3) L-sided S_3.

Cause: Cardiomyopathies or valvulopathies involving L heart.
The heart works as syncitium hence predominantly nocturnal
symptoms of LVF progress to RVF - congestive cardiac failure.
Chronic lung congestion leads to PHT, consequent RVH and
eventually RVF.

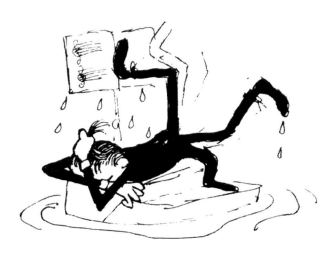

TROPPO DOLOROSO
Systemic oedema ~ RIGHT ventricular failure

Fewer symptoms, more signs of congestion

Symptoms: Patient usually 'comfortable' at rest (unless in Biventricular Failure and short of breath).

Signs: (1) Pedal oedema, (2) raised JVP, (3) hepatomegaly, (4) Ascites. Anasarca = pleural + pericardial + peritoneal effusions. (5) R-sided S_3 ventricular gallop 'distress' rhythm – 4th LICS.

Cause: L heart causes + 'C' diseases overloading R heart:

1 **C**yanotic congenital heart disease.
2 **C**or pulmonale = RVH 2° to chronic lung disease or PTED.
3 **C**lot - pulmonary thromboembolic disease.

Hypertension

Causes can be 1°, 2°, or 'malignant'.

Observation Are there clinical signs that suggest 2°HT?
Most patients have **1°HT** as part of a **metabolic syndrome**.

Roentgen and imaging
CXR: LVH, prominent calcified and unfolded aortic knuckle.
Heart, renal + adrenal U/S- may pickup suprarenal phaeo mass.
Renal artery Doppler as part of a 2°HT workup.

Diagnostic *Who to screen for possible 2°pathology?*
(1) Young person, (2) BP resistant to Rx, (3) HT of recent onset.
ECG evidence of LVH: L axis deviation and voltage criteria.
Routine bloods include renal function, low K^+ may alert to
Conns. Look for metabolic risk factors associated with HT.
Hormones - Se-aldosterone, cortisol, catecholamines, PTH.
24 hr urine collections to exclude endocrine causes.

Increased peripheral arterial resistance
HT predisposes patient to **accelerated atherosclerosis** which
causes a weakness in the vessel wall - hence strongly associated
with ischaemic heart disease and stroke, or bleed due to direct
HT- effect. Other complications include HT heart disease -
LVH as L Ventricle contracting against resistance, HT heart
failure, abdominal aortic aneurysm, retinopathy (silverwiring,
tortuous vessels, bleeds, papilloedema), HT nephropathy
(nephrosclerosis).

Strategy for anti-hypertensive therapy A B C D :
ACE-Inhibit, **B**eta-block, **C**alcium-channel block, **D**iurese.
+ **E**xtra in exceptional cases, e.g. methyldopa.
Lifestyle changes & modifiables - aspirin, lipid-lowering Rx.

HT-uncontrolled- Exclude 2°causes- 2°HT workup.

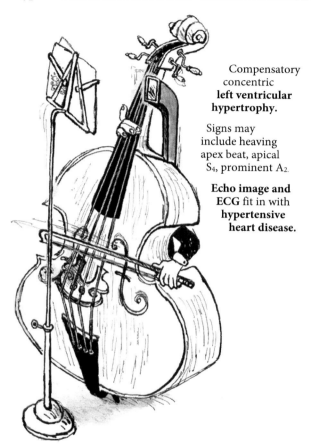

Compensatory concentric **left ventricular hypertrophy.**

Signs may include heaving apex beat, apical S_4, prominent A_2.

Echo image and ECG fit in with **hypertensive heart disease.**

THE DOUBLE BASS (A LEFT-HANDED PLAYER)

Investigate if BP not controlling - consider 2°causes:

1 **Endocrine** - **hyper**-cortisolism, -aldosteronism[1],
   - adrenalism (phaeochromocytoma)

2 **Renal impairment** - check **kidney function** routinely.

3 **Renal A. stenosis** - check for abdo renovascular **bruit**.

4 **Signs of vasculitis** - **a pulseless disease** such as **Takayasu's**
   may be diffuse or focal e.g. an **absent** radial pulse in 1 arm
   and an absent carotid pulse. Check for **bruits** over major
   vessels. **ESR↑. Angiogram** to visualize arteries may show
   multiple constrictions and aneurysms. Immunosuppressant
   Rx if life-threatening.

5 **Co-arctation of aorta** - Palpate for radio-femoral delay!

All pulses palpable? Checking all pulses will remind you to
consider a congenital or acquired **vascular** disease.

Malignant HT is **an accelerated phase** of life-threatening
end-organ damage in the presence of severe (1° or 2°) HT;
(1) Encephalopathy-fresh flame-shaped fundal haemorrhages,
brain bleed(s), (2) acute heart failure, (3) rapidly deteriorating
renal function, (4) red blood cell fragmentation.

   Patients compromise - survival is poor if untreated.
   'BP was 200/ now 150/ before I had a stroke...'

[1]**CONN'S** Consider **1° hyperaldosteronism in every case of**
HT that does not look essential.

Often goes undiagnosed.

Not responding to common anti-HT Rx.

Normally picked up on a low K+.

Serum-aldosterone ↑.

Adrenal cortex adenoma confirmed on abdominal scan.

   Rx Spironolactone is anti-aldosterone, corrects hypokalemia
until curative **surgical** adrenalectomy of the affected adrenal
gland is performed - thereafter less need for BP drugs.

   Conn's is a surgically correctable cause of HT.

A raised JVP
Where does the wave form of the neck vein originate?

1 **Pulsatile? Tricuspid incompetence**
If you see a **pulsating wave in engorged neck veins,** i.e. prominent cv waves, an unmistakable sign for **TI**; diagnoses the whole picture for you - implies there is R-sided 'congestive' heart disease and failure e.g. long-standing CMO, mitral valvulopathy or cor pulmonale 2° to COPD, ILD, or pulmonary arterial disease.

    Tricuspid valve regurgitation produces a pansystolic murmur, similar to mitral incompetence, best heard in tricuspid area 4th L ICS. It becomes louder on inspiration.

    We use external jugular vein in practice to 'read' the internal jugular venous pressure. The pulsation is accentuated by abdomino-jugular reflux. As the tricuspid valve is the last 'safety' valve, tricuspid regurgitation exerts significant pressure on the congested liver contributing to **ascites.** *A Pulsating JVP and liver is characteristic of TI.*

2 **Paradoxical? Kussmaul's sign**
Thin pencil vein that rises on deep **inspiration** may indicate **constrictive pericarditis** or big **pericardial effusion/ tamponade** which inhibits venous return.
Dyspnoea, pericardial rub, **muffled heart sounds.**

    On CXR – 'cardiomegaly' – globular with sharp cardio-phrenic angles - looks like a balloon filled with water. **Echo**-diagnosis made in a flash - fimbriae or thickened pericardium? **TB pericarditis.**

3 **Fixed? Superior Vena Cava Obstruction**
Almost all due to bronchus Ca compressing the SVC.

    Thick non-pulsating neck vein/s; Distended chest wall veins, and arm veins that do not collapse on elevation; later congestion of face and neck.

4 **COPD/ Acute asthma.**

Congenital heart disease in adults

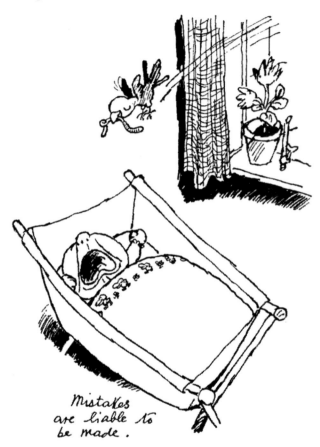

Mistakes are liable to be made.

A heart murmur - Consider congenital heart lesion.

Causes - Essentially there are two types:

1 'A'cyanotic: ASD, VSD, PDA

Initially patient is pink as the shunt flow is uni-directional from higher pressure in the Left ➜ Right. With progression of disease pulmonary vascular pressure exceeds systemic pressure. **Shunt reverses direction R ➜ L = Eisenmengers. PHT develops, patient becomes blue.** Septal defects present late when stigmata of cyanotic congenital heart disease noticed– murmur (turbulent flow - thrill), central cyanosis, clubbing.

2 **Cyanotic: 5 T's (e.g. Tetralogy of Fallot)**
            + 2 E's (Ebstein, Eisenmenger)

O/E **How to identify?** Left parasternal heave, loud P_2.
  PDA - machinery murmur maximal over pulmonary area.
  ASD - a fixed split S_2 + pulmonary flow murmur.
  VSD - harsh pansystolic murmur, lower L parasternum.
  TOF = VSD (+ Pulm. Stenosis + overriding aorta + RVH).
  Ebstein anomaly – Tricuspid valve is low-set, atrializes RV.

Roentgen chest

Diagnostic Echo differentiates shunt from valvular lesion.
            ECG helpful - RV strain pattern in V_1 /V_2.

Impending risks Pulmonary HT, big R heart; RVH-dilatation - RHF. IE, stroke 2° paradoxical emboli in ASD, arrhythmia.

Strategy for surgery
Crucial to close defect e.g. ASD or VSD repair before lungs are damaged and consequent PHT develops.

NB: SBE prophylaxis for operation or dental work.

Decades later, at an Adult Cardiology clinic:
'You've got a hole in the heart. The right and left (sides) are communicating. The hole will need to be closed which means surgery'. The problem may be picked up early - a murmur from birth. Sometimes we see a late presentation in an adult.

Acute Rheumatic Fever

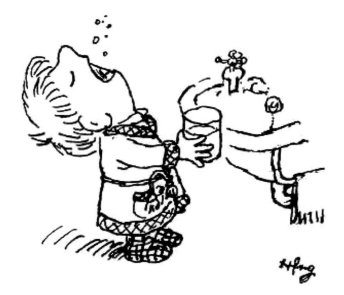

It starts with a strep throat ... sore joints ... sore heart

Mostly young patient presents with heart failure and sore joints.
Flitting 'jumping' polyarthritis picture may be quite dramatic.
Is Anti-Steptolysin O titre↑? You have a marker!
This is not viral myocarditis but acute rheumatic **pancarditis**
which requires proper REST and future vigilance.
The emphasis is on not missing the diagnosis - the infection
must be treated. Minimal residual compromise is possible after
a mild rheumatic panmyocarditis but on repeated attacks,
scarring occurs, which gives rise to nasty valvular lesions, i.e.
the valvulopathies of chronic rheumatic endocarditis.

Cause? An immune-mediated inflammation of the heart and big joints following on **streptococcal pharyngitis.** Few patients give history of prior RF, tonsillitis or sore throat.

O/E Fever and **signs** of an **acute pancarditis:**
Myocarditis = dilated heart with S_3 ventricular **gallop** rhythm.
 Endocarditis = **murmur** usually of mitral regurgitation.
 Pericarditis = central chest pain, **pericardial friction rub.**

Roentgen CXR - cardiomegaly, lung oedema?

Diagnose using Jones criteria:
Major: carditis, polyarthritis, chorea, skin lesions.
 Minor: fever, arthralgia, infective markers. Previous RF.
 Prove a preceding streptococcal infection
 ⊕ ***Throat swab* or high (and rising) ASO titre.**

Impending risks
Heart failure, mural thromboses, systemic embolization and infarction, recurrent acute on chronic rheumatic valvulitis, IE.

Strategy for **Rx** High dose salicylates, penicillin,
± cortisone for pericarditis. Rx HF - furosemide + digoxin.

How do we prevent RF? Discharge patient on RF prophylaxis - long-term daily or monthly penicillin.

How do we prevent IE - what we most fear! **Antibiotic cover** for invasive procedures - op, pre-& post-dental Rx.

Rheumatic fever pancarditis:
Infection/inflammation of all three layers of the heart.

How do you know your patient has infective endocarditis?

Causes of endocardial valve infection:
Subacute endocarditis - on abnormal valves
   SBE is a complication of chronic rheumatic valvulitis, or congenital heart lesions. Organism is mostly strep.
   Less common predisposing factors are a calcified aortic valve and prosthetic valves.

Acute R-sided endocarditis - on a normal valve
   Occurs where staph focus exists e.g. $2°$ to osteomyelitis or i.v. drug abuse; big vegetations can perforate valve. Some are fungal.

O/E suspect in presence of
   fever bacteremia? + *murmur* vegetations?

Roentgen CXR - **cardiomegaly.**

Diagnosis based on Duke's criteria
N.B. the two major being:
   $\oplus$ *Blood cultures plus*
   $\oplus$ *Echographic evidence of vegetations*

Impending risk of heart failure
Destruction of valve and heart structure, dysrhythmia, cerebral septic emboli, lung abscesses in R-sided staph endocarditis.

Strategy for Rx
Broad spectrum i.v. antibiotics - adjust according to microbial sensitivity. Refer for surgery if poor response to medical Rx, i.e. vegetations increasing in size, deteriorating heart failure.

   Systolic murmurs are graded on loudness (/6).
   Diastolic murmurs are graded on length (/4).

HEAR A HEART MURMUR?
?? Cause - What etiology do you suspect?

➤ congenital heart lesion

➤ structural valve disease

➤ functionally incompetent valves in a myopathic heart

➤ *physiological systolic flow murmur* innocent 2° to anemia

Acoustics is a difficult subject which involves distinguishing much murmuring because our ears are so untrained. Persistence pays off. Never be in a hurry, never force a diagnosis. If you find **a murmur** be patient – do **Echo to exclude a structural lesion.**

The temperature is up *and* patient has a heart murmur:

A fever must alert you. Be vigilant. Subtle signs – anemia, tachycardia - must motivate you - you may be picking up something significant. Check for immunologic phenomena such as clubbing and palpable spleen (immune hyperplasia).
SBE peripheral signs e.g. splinter haemorrhages are infrequent.

Consider immune-complex GN. Test urine for haematuria.
Echo + Blood cultures provide proof of valvular vegetations.

?Infective endocarditis
⊕ murmur ⊕ fever ⊕ anemia
makes the diagnosis likely

Helping manoeuvres to elicit an inaudible or soft murmur:

➤ **Light exercise** or change in position **enhances** murmur.

➤ **Squatting diminishes** systolic murmur in HOCM, MVP.

Mitral valve stenosis

Cause Consequence of **chronic rheumatic valvulitis.**
Be prepared to diagnose MS before ± *rumble* is heard!
MS is notoriously silent! Be open to this possibility.

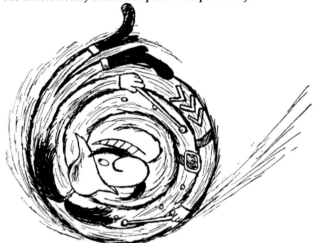

A DRUM-ROLL

O/E *Consider the suggestive 'overtones' of MS ... easy to miss.*

➤ Symptoms of **pulmonary oedema and palpitations.**

➤ Mitral facies (patient may be blue).

➤ Low volume pulse, **A**trial **F**ibrillation common.

➤ **Non-displaced tapping apex beat.**[1]

➤ **L parasternal heave** in keeping with **RVH.**

➤ **Feel apical vibration thrill** - like a **'purr'.**

---

1   Normal-sized LV 'caresses' examiner's fingertips.
    Tight MV impedes LV inflow, so LV outflow becomes fixed.
    If LV displaced - expect mixed mitral valve disease - MS/MR.

➤ **Palpable P₂ = PULMONARY HYPERTENSION.**
➤ **Loud S₁** = loudness equates severity of LA pressure.
➤ **Loud P₂** (the loud closing of valve).
➤ **Try to elicit a diastolic (murmur) rumble.**

To accentuate the murmur, turn patient leftwards to bring MV closer to chest wall, then gently rock patient from side to side; Hear apical low-pitched diastolic rumble with stethoscope bell.

The high Left atrial pressure forcing blood through narrowed orifice may produce **low-pitched** bass sound and palpable thrill.

R̄oentgen CXR Enlarged R heart.
Large L atrium causes mitralization (straight L border) of the heart, splaying of the carina and also the double shadow.
Prominent pulmonary - vasculature, trunk (PHT), oedema.

D̄iagnostic echo MV Area<1cm² is critical.
Diff diagnosis – ASD or atrial myxoma.

Īmpending risks Why is a tight MV so dangerous?
An anterograde restriction of left ventricular filling (a failure of delivery, not really a pump failure - LV myocardium is spared -underfilled and under-utilized).
An increased retrograde left atrial pressure mimics LVF. Severe **chronic pulmonary congestion** leads to **brown induration of the lungs, haemopytysis, PHT, RVH, RVF.**
There is a tendency to early symptomatic **AF palpitations.**

S̄trategy for Rx
Infective endocarditis prophylaxis (MS < MR risk).
Symptomatic diuretic therapy ↓ lung congestion.
Control rate of AF to↑ LV filling time.
Anticoagulate patient as mural thrombus can form in the stasis created by expanded left atrium. Shooting emboli cause **stroke.**
A thromboembolic event may lead to diagnosis of MS.
Surgery for symptomatic patient before PHT develops.

Aortic valve stenosis

[C]ause **Congenital:** bicuspid valve calcifies early and heavily.
    Acquired: rheumatic valvulitis, degenerative calcification.

[O]n examination
Classic signs: **heaving apex beat, feel thrill over aortic valve**
2nd R I C Space, a **rough** ejection systolic murmur - high-energy
and low-pitched - in right parasternum that **radiates to neck.**
Although aortic sclerosis is usually haemodynamically
insignificant it can produce a systolic high-pitched murmur that
radiates to apex (Gallavardin phenomenon sounds like MR).

[*PS is very much like AS. RVH, evidence **over pulmonary
valve** 2nd LICS - palpable thrill, +P_2, harsh ejection systolic
murmur that radiates to L shoulder. ECG: RV strain.*]

[R]oentgen C X R 'coeur en sabot' wooden shoe.

[D]iagnostic **Echo** - thick echogenic aortic cusps, L V H.

[I]mpending risks
Coronary ostia arise above aortic valve so angina is common.
    A I . I E . L V H . L V F. Arrhythmia. Sudden unexpected†.

[S]urgery Symptomatic patient, high pressure gradient.

**How do these patients present? (Syncope, angina, dyspnoea) -
these 'S A D' symptoms reflect cerebral and cardiac ischaemia.**

A palpable thrill over the aortic valve is pathognomonic of
tight AS. Patient looks fine. Be on your guard for this outflow
obstructive lesion - a dangerous situation. A S is insidious.

How do you pick it up? On Echo.
Chest pain - obtain Echo! Exclude aortic stenosis

Mitral valve regurgitation

The pansystolic murmur reflects regurgitant (sluggish) backwash of blood from L V to L A through an **incompetent M V** that offers low resistance to flow. MR lesion produces a constant 'to-ing and fro-ing yo-yo' **high pitched murmur.** Is apex beat displaced? We **expect L V to be large** with an **incompetent valve** (i.e. mitral or aortic). Big L A, L V result.

Cause of mitral valvulopathy - functional or structural:
> **Functional** - 2° to ring dilatation in a C M O.
> **Structural** - Rheumatic H D, I E, floppy valve. **Collagen disease** e.g. Marfan (compatible bodily features include arm span > height, lax joint ligaments, heart valves and vessel walls).
>> **Consider unusual causes: H O C M** (L V H); or
>>> **Rupture of chordae** in acute M I or I E.

Observation of severe M R
L V +. Displaced apex beat. S_1 **soft** as cusps do not co-apt. S_3.
> **PAN**systolic murmur loudest over apex spreads to L axilla.

Roentgen of chest Reveals 4-chamber cardiomegaly.
> C X R: sagging breast sign of LVH

Diagnostic Echo

Impending risks **LV dilatation, L A dilatation** but good blood flow (not static reservoir like MS) so thrombus not formed. **A F.** P H T, R V H, T I, **CCF** (heart works in high gear-heart fails); **Infective endocarditis.**

Strategy for **Rx** SBE prophylaxis. CCF symptom relief.
> Consider MV surgery early before LV (and LA) dilate.

High-pitched murmur = low energy regurgitant flow
v. Low-pitched murmur = high energy stenotic flow.

Aortic incompetence

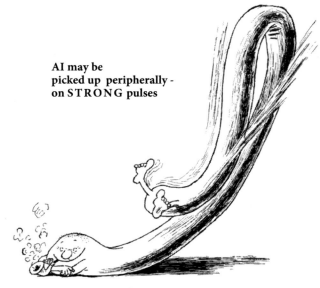

AI may be
picked up peripherally -
on STRONG pulses

A GLISSANDO

Causes of AI

Structural i.e. valvulopathy:

1 **Congenital** bicuspid valve.
2 **Acquired** - rheumatic, endocarditis.
3 **Collagen** media disorder e.g. Marfan's.

or

Functional i.e. aortic root dilatation:

1 **Hypertensive heart disease.**
2 **Aortic dissection** - severe HT, trauma, coarctation.
3 **Infective** - Rule out 3° syphilitic aortitis.
4 **Inflammatory** - large vessel vasculitis - Takayasu's.

Hand on the pulse

A big volume, collapsing, waterhammer pulse, which means **wide pulse pressure.** The wider the **pulse pressure**, the **more severe** the aortic insufficiency.

Striking *peripheral hyperdynamic signs* such as Corrigan's carotid pulsation, femoral pistol shots and strong popliteal and foot pulses are due to a big difference between systolic and diastolic blood pressures.

Hill's sign grades severity of aortic regurgitation. It is +ve if systolic B P in legs is at least 20 mm Hg higher than in the arms.

The dilated aortic root offers low resistance to blood flow- a large volume flows out and a precipitous drop is followed by a correspondingly large return flow.

Systolic B P high as heart pumps really hard to force blood out. **Diastolic B P low** as heart wants to accept and draw as much blood as possible back - both ends of scale compensate for disequilibrium.

L V enlargement- laterally and inferiorly displaced apex beat; L V size increases as regurgitated blood overloads it with each contraction.

The *early* **murmur** reflects the **forward and backward regurgitant flow** of blood inter LV and aorta through the incompetent aortic valve. **Low resistance to flow produces high-pitched murmur.** It is a central diastolic decrescendo murmur radiating down L parasternum, accentuated on leaning forwards.

(Note: systolic component sometimes present).

Roentgen chest A big 'left ventricular' heart.

Diagnostic Echo

Impending risks Enlarging heart, AF, HF, PHT, IE.

Strategy for Rx Valve surgery as symptoms develop.

Structurally incompetent valves are prone to infective endocarditis. Without much turbulence, there is time for bacteria and fibrin to settle and vegetations to grow.

Clarifying collapse ...*Dizziness* ... *'I fell down'*

O/E **?Cause** History - e.g. Chest pain, palpitations. Risks?
  CVS - P, BP, aortic stenosis murmur; carotid bruit?
  CNS - GCS Conscious? Moving all limbs, focal sign?

Routine bloods + *glucose! Troponin, D- dimers.*

Dysrhythmic pulse & ECG? *Consider 24 hour tape.*

Imaging + *cardiac work-up. Stroke work-up.*

Sudden *loss of consciousness related to?*

?Syncope *due to drop in* cerebral perfusion. **Quick recovery of consciousness.**	**?Seizure** *due to electrical discharge of brain neurons.* **Slow recovery of onsciousness.**
1 *Cardiac or CVS cause* **Exclude heart lesion e.g.** **MI** **Dysrhythmia** - fast, slow **Outflow obstruction** - stenosis of aortic valve or carotid artery. **Pulmonary embolus**	The neurons have exhausted themselves metabolically and need a prolonged post-ictal recovery phase. **EEG** **?1°/ 2° seizure**- CT scan to elucidate the diagnosis
2 *Non-cardiac cause* **Low** BP, Hb , O_2 **Metabolic** glu, K^+, thyroid Vasovagal Medication Postural hypotension **Infection** -vasodilation	*Major stroke (sudden loss of consciousness)* → *patient may not regain consciousness* → *COMA*
3 *? TIA*	

A THUD

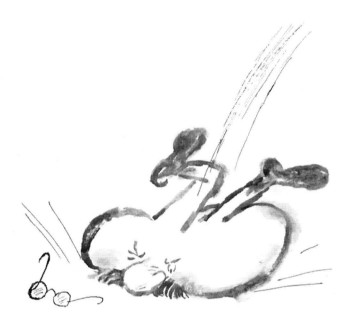

Sudden Collapse   ?Fit v. ?Syncopal attack *where drop in cerebral perfusion causes brief 'blackout' of consciousness.* When down, patient rapidly regains consciousness and a clear sensorium.

Causes of bradycardia *Pulse<60*

1 **Drugs** - digitalis, beta-blocker, calcium-channel blocker.
2 **Degenerative heart disease.**
3 **Infiltrative** - rare "…osis" eg amyloid, iron.
4 **Intracerebral pressure** ↑- Cushing reflex = ↑ BP, ↓P.
5 **Metabolic** - h**ypothyroid**, hypothermic coma - ECG monitor.
6 **Toxic**- organophosphate poisoning.
7 **O₂↓ Acute myocardial ischaenia** - risk for heart block.
   Limb leads II, III, AVF- Inferior RV wall infarction.
Hypotension - bradycardia syndrome - R coronary A. supplies SA and
AV nodes. So AV nodal ischaemia and 2° conduction block might need
temporary pacing.
8 **Physiological fitness - pulse<60**

O/E Slow heart rate palpated at the pulse.
If patient, you may view a **Cannon ball wave** in neck - a rare sighting
caused by incidental synergistic contraction of R atrium and ventricle.

Routine bloods Exclude 2° causes- TFT, Dig level.

Diagnostic ECG - is this a heart block? **Check ECG rhythm** to identify
the type of AV block. Is this a 3rd degree or **complete Heart Block**
where there is **complete loss of synchrony between atria and ventricles
with each firing at their own constant rates**?

Impending risks - exercise provokes syncope as heart rate cannot
keep pace with the exercising muscles. The slow inherent ventricular
rhythm is unable to respond and compensate for the bradycardia.
Low cardiac output. **Dizziness**. Sick sinus - arrest.

Strategy for Rx according to cause

Post-pacemaker: 'The beat was 30'
'Dr said my heart was too slow. Now, If I walk, I walk'.
Pacemaker for symptomatic Type 2 or 3° heart block.
Patient benefits from advances in modern medicine.

Coma (Gk.sleep) GCS↓ Patient not responding

Organic: Are there focalizing signs?

Metabolic and **toxic** (Kussmaul breathing suggestive)

Approach: Organic v. metabolic etiology

Cardio-Pulmonary Resuscitation in an adult

Pulse? NO PULSE.
      Call for **DEFIBRILLATOR**.
      Commence **CPR.**
CHEST COMPRESSIONS move blood. Pump heart.

Resus trolley. O$_2$ mask. Open **AIRWAY**. Simultaneous
bagging with Ambu bag while another **compressing chest.**

SHOCK VENTRICULAR FIBRILLATION
Repeat CPR for 1 minute.
Check Pulse. If no pulse – **Asystole - Adrenalin**.
Continue CPR cycles x....

'Patient stopped breathing.'
   O/E: Pupils fixed and dilated, absent corneal reflexes,
no central pulses, no spontaneous respiration, no breath
sounds, no cardiac sounds auscultated.
Requiescat in Pace.

ALL THE CAUSES - AN ANATOMICAL APPROACH

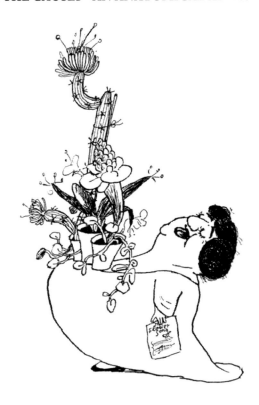

This time it was the heart. It could have been anything.
They considered a vast array of causes and excluded the dangerous ones. I have developed a way of walking slowly … a gentle walk. **Stable angina pectoris - pain responds to nitrate (gives me a headache) versus unstable angina which crescendos and is relieved neither by rest nor nitrate.**

Chest pain *Tell me about this pain*
Patient will describe -
   Position
   Area
   Intensity
   Nature- musculoskeletal pain is usually localized to chest wall,
pleuritic pain, pericarditis pain is relieved on leaning forward,
exacerbating & relieving factors. Background history. Habits.
   Does it sound…CARDIAC or Non-CARDIAC ?

O/E **Age, risk profile and Clinical presentation.**
Infarction of RV (inferior): hypotension - bradycardia.
              LV (anterior): pulmonary oedema.
Well-looking youngster, palpitations, Marfanoid features, click?
Are there **cardiac** or **lung** or **abdo** signs? Check calves for **DVT**.
Often the examination is 'normal'.

Roentgen **CXR** May indicate the cause e.g. bone pain.

Diagnostic Work-up is appropriate to the case and the risk.
?ECG: Thrombolyse hyperacute ST segment elevation MI.
Anticoagulate with Heparin other **acute coronary Syndromes**
(including unstable angina). A normal ECG does not exclude
acute ischaemia until the confirming biochemical evidence of
myocardial damage arrives.
LV dysfunction dictates heart failure therapy.
O_2, aspirin, nitrate, analgesia, b blockade, ACE-I, statin.
Unstable patient - pain, dysrhythmias→ Coronary Unit.
   Always check Troponin + D-dimers for completeness sake.
   As indicated –Echo, lung scan, or gastroscopy.

Impending risk *We all know what chest pain means!*

Strategy for **Rx** According to pathology e.g. anti-anginal.

Err on the side of caution. Exclusion of life-threatening
pathologies is a must - **acute MI, pulmonary embolus** and
aortic dissection - where pain may radiate to the back.

Causes of atrial fibrillation

1 **Structural HD** - any cardial layer or conduction system.
2 **Hyperthyroidism.**
3 **Digitalis toxicity.**
4 **Pulmonary embolus** Acute R atrium dilatation.
5 **COPD** - Chest infection can precipitate new onset AF and thence HF.

'The doctor in the cardiology unit thinks the irregular beat was occasioned by the chest infection, and there is no sign of it now.'

Observation
Symptoms Palpitations, LVF. (AF may be paroxysmal)

Signs A pulse that is irregular in volume + rhythm and an irregular heart beat with varying intensity of heart sounds. As some heart contractions are too weak for pulsations to reach the peripheries, a pulse-deficit exists between the heart & peripheral pulses.

Diff. diagnosis: Ventricular ectopics are difficult to distinguish clinically from rapid or slow AF, although here the pulse and heartbeat are only occasionally irregular. ECG needed- uni or multi-focal VEs.

Roentgen CXR

Diagnostic arrhythmic ECG
AF Baseline is 'jagged' - no P waves, QRS complexes irregular.
Atrial flutter saw-tooth baseline with 2:1 block.

Echo - **exclude** underlying structural heart lesion e.g. HT or ischaemic CMO, Cor pulmonale, **Mitral Stenosis** - **big LA** and PA pressure.

Impending risks
Systemic embolization from heart (check peripheral pulses).
Circulatory insufficiency.

Strategy for Rx
Diurese heart failure.
Find cause – Check TFT, dig level.
Control rate (± rhythm). Anti-coagulate.
Aim for rate control (especially in chronic disease).

Is the AF of cardiac or of thyrocardiac origin?
Remember conditions that strain the R heart.

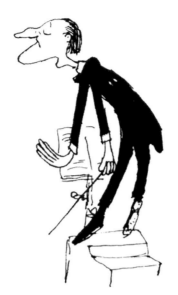

RALLENTANDO - *SLOW DOWN FAST AF*
- **ATRIAL FIBRILLATION**

Rate control - Digoxin
  If unsuccessful - add verapamil, beta- blocker.
      v.
Rhythm control - Amiodarone – good preventer.

Electrical cardioversion indicated in the decompensated patient after failed anti-arrhythmic therapy. AF may revert to sinus rhythm.
Anti-coagulate to prevent stroke.

Check thyroid function in all cases of AF.

On ECG a medley of rhythms is common in the elderly patient: sinus rhythm, atrial ectopics, AF, ventricular ectopics.

What is shock?

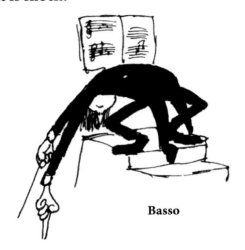

Basso

Circulatory failure irrespective of cause:
    Hypovolemia is the **no. 1**
    Haemorrhage
    Sepsis
    Cardiogenic
    Anaphylactic
    Endocrine

O/E Patient presents in shock picture…in extremis.
The main feature is **low BP**. Urine output declines steadily.

Roentgen chest may indicate underlying cause.

Diagnostic *Appropriate bloods* e.g. culture pre-antibiotics, D-dimers to exclude acute pulmonary thrombo embolus. **ECG**.

Impending risks Hypoxia & metabolic acidosis lead to multi-organ failure- deterioration of renal, liver, respiratory, cerebral functions-particularly in the elderly-underlying atherosclerosis.

Strategy for **Rx** Improve tissue perfusion!

While you support circulation with i.v. fluids - address cause:

➤ **Hypovolemic** - replace fluid.

➤ **Haemorrhagic** – volume expander, compat, transfuse blood.

➤ **Septic shock** - control infection e.g. pneumonia.

➤ **Myocardial pump failure** - post-MI or end-stage HF carries a high mortality. Infuse inotrope to improve cardiac contractility.

➤ **Anaphylaxis** - adrenaline, corticosteroid, antihistamine, O_2.

➤ **Addisonian crisis** - dextrose saline rehydration, corticosteroid.

Everything works in concert

Common emergencies

Agile conductor knows the music.

➤ **Hypoglycemia.**

➤ **Acute pulmonary oedema** Sit, O_2, i.v. furosemide, ± morphine.

➤ **Asthma** Bronchodilator nebulisers, corticosteroid, aminophylline.

➤ **Shock unstable rhythm** – but complete heart block needs pacing.

➤ **Seizures** Benzodiazepine, loading dose phenytoin if continuous.

➤ **Life-threatening** Haemoptysis - adrenalin nebs, morphia/codeine.
Epistaxis - Foley's catheter after failed nasal plug.

It's time we took a tea break!

7 THE NEPHROLOGISTS

General impression - **Vitals chart** and **Basics**
Decreased level of consciousness - acidotic breathing?

A high BP - which may be the only abnormal finding - must alert you to Renal HT. **Chronic renal failure** is difficult to pick up clinically; Consider in every case of HT, anemia, oedema.

Renal examination
Hypertensive heart disease?   Kidneys ballotable?

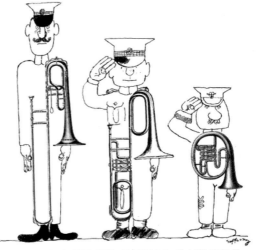

APPROACH TO RENAL FAILURE:
Is it pre-renal, renal, post-renal?
Every patient investigated gets a **U+E+creat.**

Renal failure is picked up on **routine U+E+creat**.

Elevated urea and creatinine brings a patient's often unsuspected renal impairment to light.

Not knowing whether the problem is **acute or chronic** may be unclear at first due to clinical and biochemical overlap.

Any condition that involves kidneys, or affects the waterworks.

Left venticular hypertrophy
Fluid overload can mimic the picture of pulmonary oedema and congestive heart failure. The patient apparently presents in 'CCF'- in reality he has CRF with $2°$ congestion.

Investigate kidney sizes and functioning
Renal ultrasound: We expect mostly normal-sized kidneys (measure~10x4cm, with clear cortico-medullary differentiation) in ARF and smaller kidneys in CRF. Larger exceptions include nephrotic causes, obstructive uropathy and strikingly large polycystic kidneys.
    Consider (1) Urine MCS, (2) creatinine clearance.

Strategy for Rx - prevention is the key
Your intervention can prevent renal damage from becoming chronic sparing emotional trauma and dialysis with view to transplant in end-stage CRF. *Good control of BP and DM* - the degenerative diseases - prevents rapid decline of renal function.
Fluid balance - In acute, give fluids. In chronic, fluid restrict. Most are managed conservatively - prevent deterioration. Control anasarca with furosemide. **Electrolyte** imbalances: K^+ binder for hyperkalemia, bicarb oral solution for acidosis. Calcium binds phosphate. Erythropoetin +iron for CRF anemia. Restrict dietary protein, salt, K^+, phosphate.
Rx complications e.g. UTI.
Dialysis - haemo for ARF; haemo or peritoneal for CRF.

ACUTE RENAL FAILURE

! *Disproportionate* rise in urea to creatinine indicates recent insult. Renal function is so sensitive.

ARF is an incidental finding usually diagnosed during hospitalization for another condition. It is ∴ an additional serious complication that commonly develops in the severely ill patient. Most cases are partly iatrogenic e.g. nephrotoxin is given while patient is fluid-deprived. Deterioration of renal function is usually due to combined insults - systemic infection compounded by dehydration and nephrotoxicity. Patient may be dry; or distressed and fluid-overloaded with anasarca.

Always aim to protect and recover kidney function.

Etiology?

Pre-renal
Hypoperfusion - shock during any complicated run. Oliguria. **Dehydration and infection** are the predominant etiologies. Responds well to **rehydration**; seen as a **reversible condition**.

Renal
1 **Acute tubular necrosis**-can develop after a **prolonged** phase of hypoperfusion and septic shock. Ischaemic kidney changes can regenerate with maintenance of fluid balance tided over time.
2 **Nephrotoxin.**
3 **Acute pyelonephritis** - T°, pyuria-white cell casts.
4 **Acute glomerulonephritis** - HT, oedema, **haematuria** - casts.
5 **Rhabdomyolysis** - trauma, malaria - dark myoglobinuria, ↑CK.
6 **Tubulo-interstitial nephritis**- rare - NSAIDs, infection, myeloma.
7 **Malignant HT**- fibrinoid necrosis + micro-infarcts.

Post-renal
Exclude a reversible urinary outflow obstruction.

Most cases of ARF originate outside kidneys, i.e. pre-renal. We always regard ARF as potentially reversible. Hypovolemia...ARF causes are mainly pre-renal.

CHRONIC RENAL FAILURE

! *Proportionate* rise in urea and creat.

↑Phosphate, ↓Calcium, ↓Hb - in line with CRF.

The presence of **anemia** is a marker of **chronicity**.

Subtle insults alter renal homeostasis - tipping the balance of a compromised kidney into poor excretion and deranged metabolites. Patient may be **uremic and asymptomatic**. Non-specific symptoms range from lethargy, anorexia, N + V + D, to more specific systemic features of the **uremic syndrome**: encephalopathic somnolence, puffy paleness, **Kussmaul** 'air hunger' **breathing**, skin frost (crystallized urea), pruritis, neuropathy, pulmonary oedema, bleeding and hiccups.

Etiology?

Pre-renal
Complicated ATN- prolonged shock - **hypovolemia.**

Renal
1 **Chronic glomerulonephritis.**
2 **Chronic pyelonephritis:** infection, TB, analgesics.
3 **Tubulo-interstitial nephritis.**
4 **Vascular**
   - **degenerative and immunological lesions**
   - **diabetic and hypertensive nephropathy**
   - Renal A.stenosis - congenital or atherosclerotic
   - malignant HT - fresh vascular damage
5 **Vasculitis** e.g. Takayasu's, Wegener's
6 **Inherited - polycystic, congenital UT disease.**
7 **Infiltration** - for example by TB, amyloid, lymphoma; **Myeloma kidney** is prone to infection. Hydrate to flush clogged tubules of light chains, calcium, urate. Allopurinol - hyperuricemia.

Post-renal
Urologist's domain - reflux, chronic PN, hydronephrosis; urethral stricture, prostate, chronic biharzia cystitis, cervix Ca.

Most cases of CRF are nephrogenic. Exclude pathology in the kidneys. The BP remains high. Check kidney function.

'It's all about balance. I can see when I retain fluid. Furosemide. I regulate it myself.'

Red urine [U-Dipstix: blood → microscopy U MC+S]

⊕ Red cells: can originate anywhere in the Urinary Tract.
⊖ Red cells ?due to beetroot or myoglobin.
⊕ **Red cell casts: equates renal disease = glomerulonephritis.**

As a general rule, macroscopic haematuria belongs to urology.
Bilharzia serology? If the non-relevant causes, e.g. menses are
excluded as also the big UTI group, then one can move to the
significant haematurias such as **acute glomerulonephritis**.
Pregnancy or recurring UTIs can expose pyelonephritis
scarring or a congenital UT abnormality.

Etiology: Infective   Non-infective

Infective	Non-infective

Bacterial- *E.coli* UTI *mostly*
Mycobacterial- Renal TB.
  Sterile pyuria. ++pus cells,
  but no growth.
Parasitic- *S.haematobium*
AGN haematuria red cell casts
  + hypertension + oedema
  (smoky oliguria).
Rapidly progressive GN
	Genital tract contamination
	Catheter trauma
	Toxin: Haemorrhagic cystitis
	Aspirin, warfarin
	Polycystic kidney: Burst cyst
	Malignancy
	Renal calculi: or crystalluria
	  - colicky loin pain, vomiting.

Diagnosis? Red cell cast i.e. GN or Red-cell haematuria?

Exclude proteinuria at bedside
Urine-Dipstix: Protein ++ nephrotic picture?
Check 24 hr U-protein excretion.
Range: Nephrotic proteinuria >3gm **or** Nephritic <3gm.

Renal biopsy is usually required in a case of suspected
glomerular disease to make the final histological diagnosis.

Renal anasarca

Examination Picture of **nephrotic condition**
   Peri-orbital + facial puffiness, generalized pitting oedema, anasarca (ascites and other body cavity effusions).
Shiny skin and stretch marks.
   ↑Albumin in U. ↓alb in blood.
   ↑cholesterol production (compensatory).

Nephrotic range proteinuria **>3gm/day**

A few causes of nephrotic syndrome
1° Idiopathic (common).
2° Known glomerulopathies include:
   a **diabetic glomerulosclerosis**
   b **infective** *viral* - HIV, Hep B - nephropathy
                bacterial - **post-strep GN**, IE, syphilis
                parasitic - bilharzia
   c **immune-complex vasculitis** e.g. lupus nephritis.
   d **infiltrative** lymphoproliferative - myeloma, amyloid.
   e **juvenile** - common etiology is minimal change GN.

Lesion causing the problem
Glomerulopathy - Injured glomerular capillaries disrupt glomerular basement membrane and initiate inflammatory proteinuria. The more severe and non-selective the **protein leak / loss** the worse the prognosis.
   Chronic wasting - not apparent as masked by tissue oedema.
Clotting - anticoagulant lost. **Opportunistic infections.**

Investigations **Renal U/S - large pale kidneys**, ascites.
   Serology - Infective and auto-immune screening.
Are antibodies ⊕ to Hepatitis, ASO, WR; ANF, ANCA, glomerular basement membrane?

Strategy for Rx - **depends on cause.**
Auto-immune nephritis = Prednisolone ± immunosuppressant saves glomeruli and kidney function. Prevent complications e.g. statin. Anti-HT when BP rises (as urea and creat rise). The more exudative the disease, the more steroid responsive it is, whilst the more proliferative the GN, the worse the prognosis. Monitor Rx response with 24hr protein excretion and creatinine clearance. Some are self-limiting, some progress to CRF.

8 THE PULMONOLOGISTS

A recap of the Respiratory system
A patient presents with respiratory symptoms:
cough, sputum, dyspnoea, chest pain, haemoptysis

General impression
Respiratory rate is the no. 1

Mouth? - Cyanosis is difficult to assess in the presence of anemia
- Candida, gingivitis.
- Herpes labialis *(Strep pneumoniae)*

Clubbing?

Chest examination
Always compare Left with Right:

Inspection: Shape, symmetry, movement. Signs of distress?
Palpation: Trachea central? A/symmetrical expansion?
Percussion: **Normal?**
Hyperresonant? COPD, pneumothorax.
Dull? Consolidation, mass, fibrosis
Stony dull? Fluid
Auscultation: Air entry? Any added sounds?

Be systematic - tap before listening

CXR please (PA+ Lat). Thank you.
Relax. ALWAYS stand back to see the whole picture.
View CXR from afar to compare both lung fields.

Tracheal shift

Roentgen CXR - helps locate intrathoracic pathology.

Air/ fluid - Big pneumothorax or effusion deviates trachea.

Ca bronchus - Same side as lesion (lung collapse).

Healing- Towards old TB fibrosis- flattening 2° to volume loss.

Emphysema - Tracheal tugging.

Always palpate trachea as part of the respiratory examination.

Spontaneous Pneumothorax
! Acute dyspnoea in a healthy young person must alert you to this possibility. It can happen at anytime. Cough ruptures bullus or pneumocoele in chronic lung disease such as TB.

O/E: Unilateral hyperresonant percussion note and absent breath sounds - check if trachea displaced.
Observe, be aware, and leave no doubt - do a CXR.

Remove intercostal drain when collapsed lung is expanded.

Tap and listen over lobes

Surface markings (of the lungs)

Posteriorly: 　 $\boxed{T4}$
        *Above - **upper** lobes.*
        *Below - **lower** lobes (most of lung area).*

Anteriorly: 　 $\boxed{4^{th} ICS}$
        *Above- **upper** lobes*
        *Below - **mid** lobes (RML + LUL lingula)*
          (i.e. breast areas - wedge into axillae)
        *Below 6th ICS - **lower** lobes.*

Tapping chest - a drumming sound - **percussion**

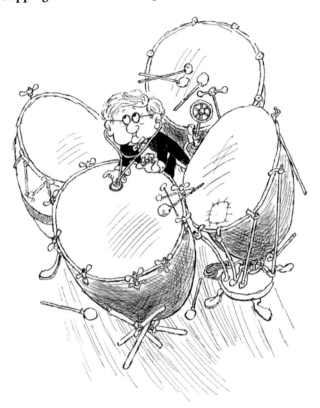

Listening to chest - a wind organ - **auscultation.**

Being systematic helps you draw out as much
information as possible.

Crepitations

Creps that clear with cough = loose secretions.
Creps that persist = fluid, infection, hypersecretions, or fibrosis.

Roentgen CXR indicates possible etiology:

Cardiac? Pulmonary? Radiological picture in keeping with heart or lung pathology e.g. cardiomegaly, or interstitial infiltrates. Marked hyperinflation or small lung volumes?

Examination signs support diff diagnosis:

Pulmonary oedema: Bibasal L H F (acute>diffuse), volume overload.
Pneumonia: Coarse creps localized to lobe(s).
COPD: Hypersecretive airways -c. bronchitis, asthma, bronchiectasis.
Interstitial lung disease: Basal or diffuse, coarse, inspiratory creps.
Cyanosis+, dyspnoea pronounced on exertion, hypoxia on blood gas.

    Causes of ILD include:

        Pneumoconiosis - asbestosis - calcified pleural plaques
        Idiopathic lung fibrosis - prominent clubbing
        Infiltrations - sarcoid, malignancy (lymphoma, Ca)
        Immunological - auto-immune

Pulmonary HT 2° to chronic lung disease.

Decreased lung compliance leads to hypoxic vasoconstriction, P H T + cor pulmonale, late-stage R H F.

Special investigations

As appropriate e.g. sputum - MCS, AFB, cytology.
Basic cardiac work up - ECG, Echo.
ABG - hypoxia.
Lung functions - may be more in keeping with obstructive FEV_1/FVC <75% vs restrictive pattern >75%.
CT lung scan to rule out ILD. Auto-antibody screen.
Consider lung biopsy if diagnosis uncertain.

Note: Deep hollow **bronchi**tis cough, chest may be clear.

Pneumonia

C̲ough Fever, shivering rigors, pleuritic pain, dyspnoea.

H̲istory Known background risk.

E̲xamination Acutely on/or **chronically ill? T°, ↑RR**
Classical signs of lobar consolidation are not always clear -area
of *dullness, ↓ air entry, crepitations, patch of bronchial breathing.*
Higher expiration note - sound is transmitted better through
dense tissue than through air; egophony say 'e' (converts to 'a'),
↑ tactile fremitus & vocal resonance. Sounds change and resolve
quickly on Rx.
Bronchopneumonia - chest noisy, scattered creps, ronchi.
CXR - lung opacification with air bronchograms = pneumonic
consolidation. Radiological & clinical correlation may be poor.
> **Obliterated anatomical borders** -
>> R Heart: R Middle Lobe pneumonia
>> L Heart: Lingula pneumonia
>> Diaphragmatic dome: Lower Lobe pneumonia.
> Lateral CXR lends more certainty - pinpoints segment/s.

**S̲ufficient admission criteria? Admit patient with poor vitals
- the 2 most important being ↑RR ↓BP**

T̲reat empirically as a **Community Acquired Pneumonia**
To improve tissue perfusion - i.v. fluids + antibiotic.
Gram+ antibiotic cover for typicals (like strep pneumoniae).

Vital signs are vital signals!
In respiratory distress? Count the respiratory tempo!
Accessory muscle usage? Intercostal recession?

Sputum - MCS, AFB + TB culture.
Naso-Gastric Aspirates - for TB
Bloods – baselines to exclude organ dysfunction.
Blood culture - T°>38^5 A life-threatening complication of
pneumococcal septicaemia is strep pneumoniae meningitis.

Picture of a poor prognostic pneumonia >1 lobe involved, ↑urea

1 *Is this a straightforward CAP?*
- **Typicals** *Strep pneumoniae is the most common bacterial pneumonia.*

2 *Does the risk profile require additional cover?*
- **Atypicals** *Legionella. Chlamydia. Mycoplasma. Serology Abs+. Mismatch between respiratory distress and the quiet lung/CXR signs.*
- **Gram negative** *Aspiration into the lungs - any predisposing reason for a depressed level of consciousness - upper lobe territory- Pseudomonas, Klebsiella. Multilobar. Poor prognostic signs. Add aminoglycoside.*
- **Anaerobic** *Binge drinker, gingivitis- Bacteroides. Add metronidazole.*
- **PTB** *Chronic pneumonia picture. Unimpressive auscultatory findings contrast with impressive CXR findings - typical apical fibro-cavitatory disease, broncho-pneumonic infiltrate and cavitation, or miliary TB.*
- **Fungal –Pneumocystis**- *Mismatch between the immunocompromised patient's 'quiet' chest and terrible tachypnoea + cyanosis.*
- **Nosocomial**

3 *Complications of pneumonia*
It is good practice to follow up all patients~1 month post-discharge for TB result and to exclude pleural effusion, empyema, abscess[1].

A non-resolving lung infection –

*Broaden diff diagnosis ?'**wrong bug**'. Test for TB.*

*Consider other organisms ?'**wrong drug**' e.g. multiple staph abscesses.*

*Consider non-infective causes ?'**complicating mechanism**' e.g.pulmonary oedema, malignant pleural effusion, Ca, lymphoma, lymphangitis, mets, pulmonary thromboemboli, drug reaction, autoimmune, rare vasculitis.*

---

1 **Lung abscess - post-aspiration** - *necrotic lung tissue breaks down and communicates with bronchus; air-fluid level/s develop - foul purulent sputum expectorated. Smell the picture of suppuration: halitosis, gingivitis + clubbing, ±amphoric (exaggerated bronchial) breathing over a cavity.*

Lateral CXR locates position of abscess. **Typical aspiration territory** *(in supine position - apex of lower lobe, or posterior segment of upper lobe). Triple therapy - metronidazole + penicillin + aminoglycoside + postural drainage physiotherapy.* **Atypical location+ no risk** *(for aspiration)-e.g. RML syndrome - consider bronchus Ca or Upper Lobe - PTB (or Gram-).*

Pleural Effusion Latin 'Effundere' = to pour out

Lung signs **Fluid - stony dullness, no air entry.**
Verify with ↓ tactile fremitus and ↓ vocal resonance.
Father of percussion - von Auenbrugger - 1st physician to tap a
chest. He implemented a technique he learnt from his Austrian
father–innkeeper–who tapped wine barrels to check their levels.

Exudate vs transudate - **Diagnostic tap**

Usually **unilateral effusions are exudative** - TB, malignancy.
      bilateral effusions are transudative - Organ failures.
Unusual causes include **auto-immune serositis** or small bloody
effusion if area of **lung is infarcted post-pulmonary embolus.**
Subdiaphragmatic pus/amebic penetration to chest, pancreatitis.

Roentgen-does the CXR concur with your clinical findings?
Meniscus? Is costophrenic angle clear?

Approach **Aspirate pleural fluid** (most are straw-coloured).
Biochemistry differentiates a **low protein** transudate from a
high protein exudate.
Further tests - **MCS, TB culture, ADA, cytology.** Securing
needle position on top of rib avoids neurovascular bundle.
Therapeutic tap indicated for respiratory distress.

    Drain empyema. Hippocrates said *'ubi pus ibi evacuo'*,
literally 'where there is pus, there I empty'. It still stands!

Take away message

The disease fits risk profile … age, smoking, asbestos exposure.
Immunosuppression raises the index of suspicion for TB.
Bronchus Ca and TB go hand in hand. 'Once the TB (effusion) was
treated the malignancy came to the fore.' Is there parenchymal lung
disease or pleural thickening? Is there clinical evidence to support the
diagnosis of lung Ca? Follow up CXR mandatory after TB Rx.
Pleural biopsy may be needed to confirm the diagnosis e.g. TB
pleuritis or mesothelioma.
A large pleural effusion is usually tuberculous or malignant.
Small exudative effusion - parapneumonic, thrombo-embolic.

*TB predilection for **membranes**: pleura- pericard- peritoneum- meninges.*

Lung Ca

$1°$ may be in **lung parenchyma, bronchus, or pleura.**

When a **heavy smoker** develops **new or worsening respiratory symptoms** take note! **A chronic cough** is the commonest finding. Bronchial Ca infiltrates and occludes the lumen causing an obstructive lung syndrome i.e. chest infection that does not respond to Rx. Most are inoperable at diagnosis. AdenoCa is less smoking-related; some originate peripherally and may be amenable to early surgery.

Usually peripheral signs more impressive than lung signs.
1 **Systemic: Wasting**
2 **Paraneoplastic: Clubbing**
3 **Metastatic: Cervical lymphnodes**
4 **Infiltrative: SVCO** - engorged fixed veins in neck + upper torso;
    Hoarse voice - paralysed vocal cord. **Horner** - ptosis, miosis.

Non-specific lung signs
Hyperinflation is the most constant finding.
    Area of dullness is suggestive of collapse/ consolidation.
    Large pleural effusion in a smoker is always suspicious.

Gathering evidence from:
CXR - Lung mass is what stands out most, bronchus 'cut-off' sign, mediastinal nodes, mets, effusion- consider concurrent TB.
Scan chest - stage disease - bony erosion, invasion of chest wall.

Blood: Paraneoplastic syndrome?

PTH-like: ↑corrected calcium - non-small cell Ca; long-standing - signs appear late.
SIADH: ↓Na, Cl, osmolarity - small cell Ca lung; aggressive - metastasizes early and widely, chemo-sensitive.

Sputum - cytology + malignant cells, **microscopy** - for TB.
Biopsy - bronchoscopy; pleura in case of malignant effusion.

As there is usually little in the way of chest signs, look at the hands of a wasted smoker and pay attention to the neck. Have you noticed hoarseness and palpated supraclavicular fossae?

Sensitivity to smoking and occupational history.

$\boxed{A}$ wheeze   Is it asthma or not?

$\boxed{S}$ymptoms **How it feels**	$\boxed{S}$igns **How it sounds**
'Tight chest. Like an airbag -air can't come in - or out. It's a battle - obstructive.'	A bronchospastic cough, a high-pitched, prolonged and dominantly expiratory wheeze.

$\boxed{T}$rigger of bronchospasm?

Acute exacerbation of asthma - Be on high alert in the CVS patient who presents with acute-onset respiratory distress and a new wheeze. Consider cardiac asthma. Exclude the unexpected: **pulmonary oedema** (cardio /nephrogenic), **embolus, infection.** *Consider other causes:* Difficult 'asthma' may not be asthma.

Allergen, e.g. smoke, aspirin. *'It attacks me immediately.'*
Allergic rhinosinusitis. Anaphylaxis. Aspiration. Airway obstruction - Stridor - ENT - laryngoscopy - for intubation?
COPD *'I got blocked through smoking-as I grew up I had no asthma'*
Carcinoid. Eosinophilic lung infiltrate. GERD.
Paediatric - worms, bronchiolitis. Secretions.

Problem:	In such a case- Investigate Bloods - Asthma profile:
Uncontrolled asthma Persistent wheezing Frequent attacks 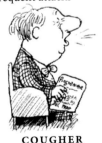 **COUGHER**	1 *Eosinophil count* 2 *ESR* 3 *ANCA* *A rare vasculitis?* 4 *IgE* ↑*Allergic / Parasitic etiology.* 5 *Aspergillus serology Allergic bronchopulmonary Aspergillosis causes central bronchiectasis with clubbing and recurring haemoptysis.* **Echo** - exclude cardiac asthma. **CXR** - heart, lung, other disease.

Lung functions - Check under stable conditions in order to assess severity, monitor Rx, clarify an uncertain case, determine reversible bronchospastic component in COPD.

Hospital admission for acute severe asthma /bronchospasm.
Consider every severe case to be life - threatening!
Err on side of caution. Stop. Count the respiratory rate.
This will sensitize you to the level of respiratory distress in a
patient that might initially appear comfortable. **Respond** to this
sub-optimal vital sign by **admitting patient. O_2.**
CXR - exclude pneumothorax.
i.v. fluid; corticosteroid ± aminophylline .
Nebulized bronchodilator inhalations almost back to back.
Re-check poor blood gas.
Laboured breathing is the warning sign of impending
ventilatory failure. Hypoxia with cyanosis and confusion,
exhaustion, severe wheeze, or silent chest when no or little air
enters (hypoventilation). Resistant **status asthmaticus** may
require non-invasive or invasive ventilation (low + pressure
prevents barotrauma from bullae rupture).
Physio - clears mucus plugs that can cause atelectasis.
Ensure adequate hydration.

Manage: Is 'asthma' really asthma? Other causes?

Asthma **is an inflammatory airways disease.**
Optimize control to prevent lung damage from intermittent or
ongoing bronchial hyperreactivity. Aim to attain and maintain
best possible lung function. Clear airways. Improve air flow.

To reduce inflammation - start high dose corticosteroids, taper.
To reduce bronchospasm / bronchial tone relieve symptoms -
with regular bronchodilator therapy: oral theophylline+
pumps[1]- *'part of my living - help to remove the secretions and
help me breathe freely and lightly. I can even run.'*

A happy patient - compliant on Rx - improved lung function.
Monitor PEF and **FEV_1 / FVC**

1Pumps: b_2 agonist ± anticholinergic ± corticosteroid.

Chronic obstructive pulmonary disease

Chronic airway inflammation Chr.bronchitis, emphysema, asthma.

    Destructive bullous disease Emphysema, old P T B, sarcoid.

    Bronchiectasis Hereditary /Acquired: clubbing, coarse basal creps.

On a mixed continuum of COPD:

Chronic Bronchitis	**Emphysema**
Centrilobular emphysema.	Panacinar
Chronic hypoxia, hypercarbia.	Hyperinflation. Pink.
Centrally cyanosed, >rotund.	Lip pursing.
Early respiratory failure.	Late respiratory failure.
Dusky Cor Pulmonale.	Lots of air, few sounds.
Noisy chest.	Quiet chest.
Chronic productive cough.	CXR- Big lung volumes,
Thick mucus in bronchi.	air-trapping, thin heart,
Big R heart, RHF common.	prominent pulmonary Aa.

Pulmonary hypertension

Prolonged inflammation of the airways leads to hyperinflation and ultimately to PHT+ cor pulmonale. A hyperinflated chest obscures the apex beat and L parasternal heaving heart - and its sounds. In cor pulmonale the RV epigastric pulsation features quite prominently.

Discharge of patient

Recover some lung function; optimize bronchodilator therapy, antibiotic for purulent sputum, diuretic for incipient RHF.

    Check ABG for hypoxia and hypercarbia. As hypoxic / CO_2 drive stimulates respiration, prescribe low concentration O_2 in COPD. Theophylline reduces pulmonary artery pressure.

    Avoid digitalis - AF risk.

    Discourage smoking.

Acute exacerbation of COPD ?Precipitant

Any insult that adds to the work of breathing plummets the patient into striking shortness of breath - chest infection, bronchospasm, pneumothorax, pulmonary emboli and heart problems such as acute MI with arrhythmia and failure.

THE TRUMPET SHALL SOUND

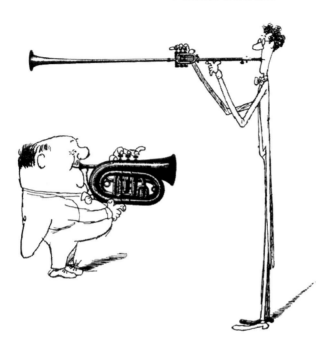

Does the patient tend to a *Blue Bloater* or a *Pink Puffer*?

Dum spiro spero - *While I have breath I have hope*

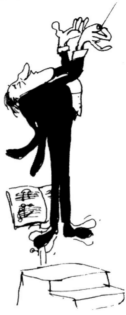

A CAPPELLA

Is the patient's chest hyperinflated? AP↑
The normal AP diameter relative to the lateral is 5:7.
In COPD this AP diameter is increased relative to the lateral approximating or exceeding 1:1 (barrel chest).
Is upper border of liver where it is supposed to be - in 5th ICS?
The liver is inferiorly displaced (percusses below its normal position in the 5th ICS MCL).
Loss of cardiac dullness i.e. the chest is hyper-resonant.
Is the patient using extra muscles to support breathing?
Decreased lateral expansion; chest moves upwards.
Poor air entry. Scattered coarse creps and wheezes are common.

Haemoptysis

Red **blood** coughed up: *False - after a nose bleed*

Etiology: **lung** Oedema[1], Infection[2], Infarction[3], Ca.

Diagnosis: chest examination + CXR

Bloods + **Sputum:** MCS, AFB + TB culture, cytology.

Do not overlook a cardiac or
acute thrombo-embolic cause.
Chest pain and dyspnoea in the presence of a rapid pulse or
fast AF and normal T° may alert you to a clot!

---

1   **Cardiogenic** frothy pink sputum e.g. **Mitral Stenosis.** Echo.

2   **Any pneumonia** –especially a **necrotizing bacterial infection** in drinkers; **TB or lung abscess** can erode a vessel and cause massive haemoptysis. **Aspergillus - invasive** lung infection in neutropenic setting. **Aspergilloma** dormant fungus ball colonizes old apical TB or sarcoid cavity. **Bronchiectasis** may cause a chronic cough productive of copious and foul sputum with recurring specks of blood. Post-necrotic pneumonia, or post-TB. Allergic Bronchpulmonary Aspergillosis (resistant wheeze leads to diagnosis)

3   **Pulmonary vessel disease - Embolus with infarction high on list.** This is a dramatic interruption - a big clot can close off pulmonary artery and infarct part or whole of lung; a blob of blood … can cause shock, severe acute **dyspnoea,** central cyanosis, RV dilatation, **acute R sided heart failure** with raised JVP, **PHT** - loud P_2 and **R**-sided S_3 gallop. A smaller clot causes **chest pain**, tachycardia, sometimes ECG and blood gas changes. Recurring small emboli cause acute episodes of chest pain. Are calves soft, equal diameter? **D-dimers↑.** **CXR** – may be inconclusive. Prominent PA trunk. Are both lungs equally perfused? Wedge-shaped pleural-based circulation defect. **Move** to diagnostic CT- angiogram. Anti-coagulation for **PTED** x 6/12. Recurrent - lifelong.

Unusual causes of haemoptysis:

   Vasculitis - Goodpasture's - haemorrhagic lung infiltrates + rapidly progressive glomerulonephritis and acute renal failure. **Wegener's.** **Angiodysplastic vessels.**

9 THE GASTROENTEROLOGISTS

Recap to get into the rhythm of systematic observation

General examination
Global overview Vitals Basics JACCOL
Put out your tongue. Let's see your eyes - look up, down.

Systematic abdominal examination

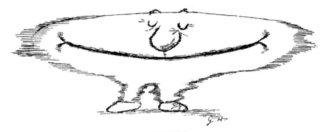

A HUM

- **Inspectio** Shape and symmetry.
- **Palpatio** Organomegaly, mass.
- **Percussio** Elicitable ascites?
- **Auscultatio** Bowel sounds.

Normal or abnormal?

Percussion tenderness = peritonism → **Surgeon**

Most gastro-intestinal medicine is related to
liver cirrhosis or to gut pathology -
domain of the hepatogastroenterologist.

Ascites of uncertain etiology

Signs Bulging flanks, smiling or everted umbilicus.
If no fluid thrill, check for shifting dullness.
Hepato-splenomegaly? (often difficult to palpate)

Can you link ascites to ORGAN FAILURE?
Heart (+its **bag**[1]) congested neck veins and liver, pedal edema.
Renal – nephrotic proteinuria - periorbital, puffy oedema.
Liver – cirrhosis - fibrosis - portal hypertension caput.
Intestinal – hypoalbuminemia - malnutrition/ malabsorption.
Thyroid – myxoedema

When you can't localize the cause for the patient's ascites...In the absence of diagnostic features to support a transudative etiology - did you consider the possibility of an exudative effusion due to:

Infection - T B peritonitis (lymphocytes,↑ADA,+TB culture).
Malignancy- ovary, lymphoma, GIT, hepatoma, mesothelioma.
Uncommon cause - pancreatitis, serositis, pus.
Blocked lymphatic or venous drainage.

Investigations Routine + serology + selected e.g. CA 125.

Tap ascitic fluid = diagnostic tap (biochem, micro, cytology).
Biochemistry - transudate v exudate (based on protein).
Relevant tests. Tender abdomen - culture fluid - SB peritonitis[2].

Excessive portal venous pressure - complication of cirrhosis

Sonar Utrasound of **abdominal organs and heart early in work-up of ascites.**

---

1 **Not to be forgotten:** Constrictive pericarditis or tamponade - Kussmaul JVP sign.
2 **Spontaneous Bacterial Infection** of transudative ascites.

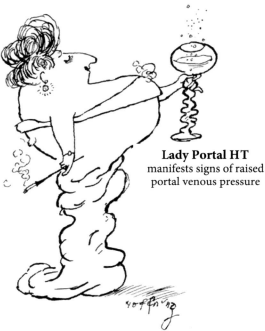

Lady Portal HT
manifests signs of raised
portal venous pressure

1 *Pronounced hepatic ascites (cf. wasted limbs).*
2 *Caput = superficial lateral abdominal wall veins.*
3 *Gastroscopic evidence of oesophageal varices.*

The liver is usually small in alcoholic & non-alcoholic **cirrhosis.**
The principal cause is alcohol. What are non-alcoholic causes?

➤ **Bilharzia: Hepatic *Schistosomiasis mansoni* infection** causes
periportal fibrosis. High portal pressure obstructs venous
drainage from the gut - hepatopetal flow is thus reversed -
portal vein dilates - splenomegaly and collaterals develop.

➤ **Chronic hepatitis B or C.**

➤ **Auto-immune** biliary cirrhosis-pruritis,↑ALP, mitochondrial abs.

➤ **Infiltrations** large cirrhotic liver - iron, fat, amyloid, copper.

$\boxed{\text{A}}$lcoholism Coarse beefy facies and parotomegaly

$\boxed{\text{L}}$iver and other systemic complications

$\boxed{\text{C}}$irrhosis Fat infiltration, toxic hepatitis, liver failure, SBP.

$\boxed{\text{O}}$esophageal varices - haematemesis.

$\boxed{\text{H}}$eart HT, 'holiday heart' dysrhythmias, beriberi and dilated
CMO. Direct and indirect cardiotoxic effect.

$\boxed{\text{O}}$ral cavity, alimentary tract and abdominal
Lower lip depigmentation. Gingivitis bacteroides reservoir +
vomitus predisposes binge drinker to aspirate from mouth.
Acute & chronic gastritis, pancreatitis.
Malnutrition, ↓VitB$_3$ = Pellagra.

$\boxed{\text{L}}$ungs Prone to aspiration pneumonia and PTB.

$\boxed{\text{I}}$ntoxication and chronic toxic neurological sequelae
Withdrawal - DT's, seizures, Wernicke's thiamine ↓vit B$_1$.
Untreated, Korsakoff's develops. Patient confabulates.
Cerebral and **cerebellar degeneration**.
Myelin damage to brain, spinal cord, peripheral nerves.
Muscle damage - myopathy, rhabdomyolysis.
Skull fracture with subdural haematoma.
Entrapment neuropathy.
Hepatic encephalopathy.
Stroke haemoconcentration.
Fetal Alcohol Syndrome.

$\boxed{\text{S}}$ocial and familial dysfunction

$\boxed{\text{M}}$etabolic and endocrine and haematological
↓Clearance of estrogen in the cirrhotic liver. **Gynaecomastia**.
Shakespeare wrote that alcohol provokes the desire but takes
away the performance. Patient becomes feminized. **Testicular
atrophy. Osteoporosis. Pseudo-cushingoid obesity**.
Sleep apnoea - tendency to snore. **Hypoglycemia, gout,
↑Triglyceride, diabetes 2° to calcified pancreas**.
Macrocytosis, hypersplenic pancytopenia, low prothrombin.

Vomiting!

Take note! Alerto! Exclude life-threatening disease.
Do not ignore this non-specific sign which may accompany a
more specific diagnostic indicator. To adopt a careful and in-
depth approach to its cause, **broaden** your etiologies. **Look
further** - DKA, myocardial infarction, malaria, gut obstruction.

Cause?

INFECTIVE	NON-INFECTIVE

Gastro-enteritis
Whilst straightforward GE is more commonly thought of, other masked problems may be overlooked. Consider **other** causes!
 	
Systemic infection
e.g. hepatitis, typhoid, pyelonephritis, malaria.
 	
Every patient deserves at least a urine dipstix.
Blood glucose↑
 	
Don't miss a potentially fatal treatable condition.
	Diet, Drugs
	Intestinal - GERD
	Ischaemic - brainstem, heart
	        - bowel, gonad
	Inflammation - peritonitis
	Intracerebral pressure↑
	Metabolic, endocrine
	        - uremia, DKA!
	        - Addisonian crisis
	Migraine or Labyrinthitis
	Toxin
	Obstruction - hollow organ
	Pregnancy
	Psychogenic - anorexia

Vomiting masks a lot of pathology that can really fox you.
    Haematemesis requires urgent gastroscopy.
    Peritonism lies in the domain of the surgeon.
Peritonitis - acute abdomen - is the final common pathway.
Erect Abdo XRay + CXR (?air under diaphragm).

Severe Diarrhoea

Cause?

INFECTIVE	NON-INFECTIVE
Gastro-enteritis spectrum ➤ **viral** common ➤ **bacterial** salmonella, shigella, clostridium antibiotic colitis, cholera rice-watery stools ➤ **mycobacterial** ➤ **protozoal** amoeba, giardia ➤ **parasitic** bilharzia. **As part of systemic infection** **HIV** - consider poly-microbial enteritis - Intestinal TB (involves ileo-caecal lymphoid tissue). **Other** - **malaria**, legionella.	**Diet, Drugs** **Irritable bowel syndrome** **Inflammatory bowel disease** **Immunologic** - scleroderma **Infiltrative** - amyloid **Malabsorption** - celiac **Malignancy** - **carcinoid** - **big liver mets** 2° to midgut 1°. ↑24hr U-5HIAA. Neuroendocrine slow-growing tumour. **Metabolic, endocrine** - Thyrotoxicosis, DM autonomic neuropathy **Toxin** - organophosphate

Obvious dehydration is only evident in children. **In adults** we are guided by a **low BP, a rapid pulse.** Skin turgor and dry tongue are unreliable signs of significant **hypovolemia** complicated by pre-renal dehydration.
Alert to fluid and potassium balance in V+D.
Vitals remain vital. Hypotension.
    Severe hypokalemia - replenish.
Plan: Stool for MC+S.
    Rehydrate.
    Empiric antibiotic cover if (bloody) **dysentery** until microbe identified – Ampicilin/ Sulphonamide/ Quinolone for **?salmonella**, Metronidazole for **amebiasis** or for antibiotic-associated Clostridium (± Vancomycin). Tetracycline and ample fluid is the secret for cholera.

Diarrhoea is a prominent manifestation of enteric infection - in contrast to vomiting - a more ominous sign.

Chronic diarrhoea

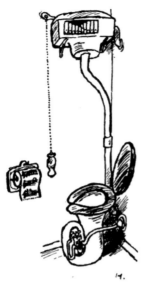

Symphonia domestica
Musical
rearrangement

Intestinal Failure? 2° to chronic pancreatic or small bowel (ileal) disease.

Maldigestion *Pancreatic*
Faecal elastase↓ = exocrine↓.

Malabsorption *Enteropathy*
Short bowel, lymphoma, Fistulae- intestinal TB, Crohn's; Celiac (biopsy, Abs).

Albumin low Oedema.
If case looks like protein-losing enteropathy refer for radiographic follow-through study / endoscopy / histology.

Loss of weight Cachexia.
Extreme weakness. Neuropathy.
Malnutrition. Nutritional support.
Supplement Calcium-Fe-folate-B$_{12}$

Constipation

Diet, drugs, dehydration.
Irritable bowel syndrome.
Metabolic, endocrine - ↑calcium, ↑TSH.
Trauma - painful anal fissure.
Organic bowel disease - change of bowel habit.
Plan - *FBC, TSH, CEA. Colonoscopy if indicated.*

Functional versus organic bowel disease?

Possible OD Contact Poison Information Centre

Observation
History
O/E- Patient conscious and responding? e.g. para-sympathetic cholinergic manifestations: hyper-secretions (sweating, wet lungs, V+ D), bradycardia, pinpoint constriction of pupils.

Identify poison Toxic screen + appropriate tests.
Low se-cholinesterase points to organophosphate poisoning.
Specific antidotes are few:
naloxone for morphine, anexate for benzodiazepines.
Acetylcysteine prevents paracetamol liver failure.

OD pills - ↓ absorption
Gastric lavage still part of the toxicologist's management (non-corrosive substances) + activated charcoal.
Admit for observation. **Supportive Rx** - fluids, complications.
Maintain O_2 saturation - ventilate if Glasgow Coma Scale low.

Neutralize the toxin at end-organ level
e.g. ethanol for methanol, and atropine for organophosphate.
  Monitor and titrate dosage against clinical picture.

AN ADD ON...ALCOHOL
Alcohol usually augments other problems.
  Loss of control, unpredictability.
  'A tot too much, A bottle not enough.'
  'All women become object of affection'.
  Risk of STDs.
  Patient becomes depressed and escapes in alcohol.

**These are the hidden hazards of
alcohol, a systemic toxin.**

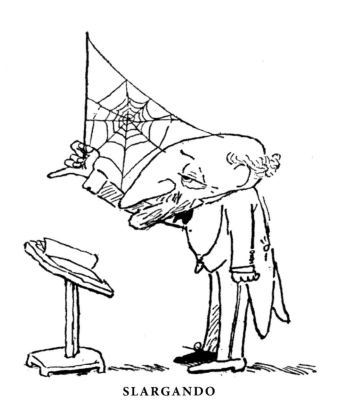

SLARGANDO

10 THE NEUROLOGISTS

General examination
Glasgow Coma Scale   Vitals and Basics

Shortened neurological examination...

A sorting out process: Observe signs. Now link to pathology.

1 **Higher functions**
2 **Meningism**
3 **Pupils**
4 **Cranial nerves** Facial asymmetry, speech
5 **Motor Weakness? L = R? Focalizing signs?**
   Upper and Lower limbs - distal and proximal
   A **Muscle bulk**
   B **Tone**
   C **Power** 0/5 plegia = paralysis, paresis = weakness
   D **Reflexes** (clonus = 4+)
6 **Sensation** Focus on area of interest
7 **Cerebellar** Co-ordination: past point = dysmetria
8 **Extrapyramidal** Rigidity + abnormal movements
9 **Gait**
10 **Include CVS exam:** Pulse regular?
   Auscultate heart, carotids

No neck stiffness
No neurological deficit
Is the patient metabolically corrected?
Do glucose routinely - bizarre hypo presentations!

Is the patient's gait and posture normal?

- ➤ **Spastic** hemi-scissor circumduction.
- ➤ **Neuropathic** sensory high-stepping foot drop.
- ➤ **Myopathic** lordotic waddle.
- ➤ **Broad based.**
- ➤ **Parkinsonian** shuffling, loss of spontaneous movements.
- ➤ **Dystonic** (walk with outer edges of feet).

Disturbance of gait – loss of balance

1 **Vertigo: 'Dizziness, giddiness'**

- ➤ **Peripheral:** Vestibular - positional vertigo excluded on history.
- ➤ **Central** - Acute brainstem features, e.g. stroke.
  - Chronic, e.g. tumour pressing on central connections.

2 **Cerebellar ataxia**

Toxic - alcohol, anti-epileptic; nutritional - $B_{12}\downarrow$; infective; metabolic-thyroid; vascular; space-occupying; multiple sclerosis; genetic - hereditary degeneration, high cervical cord syrinx + cerebellar herniation.

Delirium Tremens or classical Wernicke's encephalopathy can be prevented in a possible drinker by adding vitamin BCo + thiamine to dextrose drip - promotes remyelinization. Benzodiazepine prevents seizures in a tremulous, agitated patient. Alcohol intoxication and withdrawal lowers seizure threshold.

3 **Sensory ataxia**

- ➤ **Severe peripheral neuropathy**
  Small fibre neuropathy = Numbness, burning feet or pins and needles.
  Large fibre neuropathy = Romberg+, loss of vibration and joint position sense.

- ➤ **Spinal cord disease** - dorsal columns.
  Syphilis - Tabes dorsalis.
  $B_{12}\downarrow$ - Combined degeneration of lateral + dorsal cord.

Movement disorders

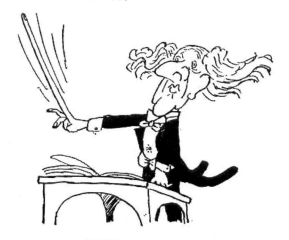

SENZA BATONE
Without baton - involuntary shaking movements

Extrapyramidal signs: ↑tone, ↑reflexes, cogwheel **rigidity**

Disease or drug affecting the Basal Ganglia:

Hyperkinesia

➤ **? Epilepsy, encephalitis.**
➤ **? Flinging - Hemiballismus** - acute onset - stroke - DM, HT.
➤ **?Chorea, dystonia picture** - jerky movements.
Drug-induced, HIV, SLE, Hereditary.
Sydenham's - major sign of acute rheumatic fever.

Bradykinesia

Parkinson's Disease	*v.*	**Parkinsonism**
Tremor asymmetrical		Tremor symmetrical
Mask facies		2°causes (drug history?)
Monotone speech		P'plus multisystem atrophy

Headache!

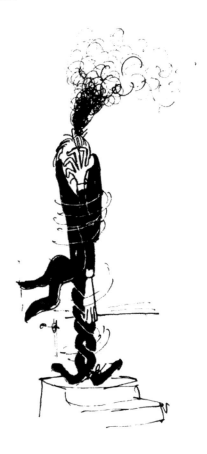

RINFORZANDO

New persistent headache not responding to analgesia.

Dangerous headache? Check *duration.*

Intracranial pressure raised?

Meningism? **Neck stiffness & T°,** delirium.

Take note of **severe progressing headache.**

Organic? **Focalizing signs.**

Plan: **Look for focalizing sign** + papilloedema- **brain scan 1st.**
   Trauma: Yo-yo consciousness ?Subdural haematoma.
Intracerebral haemorrhage: Sudden thunderclap headache -
the like of which the patient has never had before…vomiting ±
collapse, loss of consciousness, neck stiffness. Exclude
subarachnoid bleed.

Picture of suspected meningitis- Do LP
CSF analysis:

Macroscopic appearance, Biochemistry (↑protein, ↓glucose & chloride),
Microscopy cell count + culture (Gram+diplococci=Strep.pneumoniae).
Bacterial antigen, Cryptococcus India Ink. ADA, Cytology on occasion.
Empiric broad spectrum antibiotic covers Neisseria/Strep pneumoniae.
Neck stiffness is an unreliable sign in immune compromise – Consider
fungal (Cryptococcus)/TB etiology (lymphocyte predominance).

Less severe headache

> **Vascular** - migraine.
> **Tension** - intermittent 'frightful headache'.
> **Inflammatory** - sinus congestion.
> **Infection** - **localized**- sinusitis.
>   - **systemic**- viral, bacterial e.g. typhoid, rickettsial, malaria.
> **Chronic** - blurred vision, papilloedema - pseudo-tumour cerebri.

The conundrum of Confusion

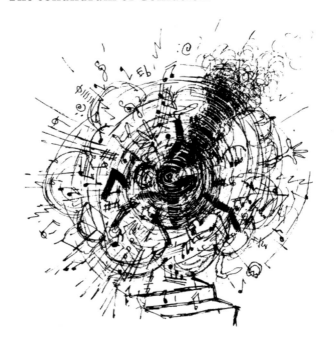

FINALE FURIOSO

Is he in a confused state? Patient is disorientated.

Etiology unknown. Did you consider all causes?

DIMTOP covers and unravels any confusion 'circuit' from
alertness through to coma.

Decreased or altered level of consciousness

Infective? Cerebral- meningitis; **Systemic** – e.g. typhoid.

Metabolic? Metabolites corrected? Organ failure?

Toxic? Drugs, alcohol: too much, too little (DTs).

Organic? Exclude intracerebral space-occupying lesion.

$O_2\downarrow$ Hypoxia e.g. pneumonia, cerebral malaria.

Post-ictal confusion?

SEIZURES

**If no metabolic or structural cause is found, exclude
1° idiopathic epilepsy. Known epileptic patient?** Epilepsy can
present in bizarre ways - motor or sensory or behavioural
changes and other autonomic phenomena such as sweating.
Urinary incontinence.
History + Collateral history. Usually starts in teens.
EEG evidence - to be safe.
Benzodiazepine stat. If the fits recur – anticonvulsant - loading
dose Phenytoin prevents or aborts a continuous '**status**' seizure;
start maintenance therapy.
Exclude **2°cause for the convulsion(s)** i.e. **provoked,** e.g. stroke.
Every 1st (new onset) seizure in an adult warrants a **brain scan.**

To pin down the etiology do a basic work-up.

*Bottom line: Restlessness or obtundation in a patient – Exclude
metabolic cause, starting with the **glucose** – the **no. 1** priority.*

Hyper-hypoglycemic seizures can confound the picture.
U + E + creat. Any obtunded patient who does not have a clear
metabolic cause needs a brain scan. Containdications to LP:
SOL on brain scan, focal neurological signs, papilloedema.

Ongoing confusion… A complete work-up breaks through the
'cloud of unknowing'. Don't dismiss a psychotic case. Have you
excluded all non-psychiatric **acquired causes** before referring
the patient for psychiatric assessment: TSH, B_{12}, autoimmune
disease, substance abuse, HIV infection, neurosyphilis, stroke,
head trauma, 1°frontal lobe tumour or 2°cerebral mets. Bear in
mind the chronic degenerative and multi-infarct dementias.

$\boxed{\text{W}}$eakness Etiology? 1st step: Is it UMN or LMN?

$\boxed{\text{E}}$licit the signs to localize the pathology.

$\boxed{\text{A}}$pproach Upper or lower motor neuron weakness?

$\boxed{\text{K}}$eep anatomical station or level in mind. Where is the lesion?

UMN disorder? *Central LESION ABOVE anterior horn cell*

1 **The Brain** *Hemiparesis* - ↑tone, ↑reflexes, pathological Babinski+. Acute flaccid shock phase; **UMN** spasticity develops later.

2 **The Spinal cord** *Paraparesis* - sphincters, motor + sensory cut-off. **Exclude compressive cord lesion.** Check **Spinal XRay for ?Trauma, Tumour** - bone mets, **TB** - gibbus. **Backache,** kyphosis 2°to vertebral collapse - Refer Spinal unit. Regard as potentially treatable - some cases can recover leg power.
   Consider a non-compressive myelopathy in the absence of a clear sensory level: hereditary spastic paraparesis; inflammatory/ infective-viral myelitis, neurosyphilis; lupus; demyelinating disease; toxic; B_{12}↓.

LMN disorder? *Peripheral LESION BELOW anterior horn cell.*

1 **The anterior horn cell** *Fasciculations* (check tongue). Motor Neuron Disease - mixed UMN+LMN signs. Cervical spondylosis - UMN signs in legs; Syrinx.

2 **The peripheral nerve** *Symmetrical distal weakness–Neuropathies* **Flaccid paralysis- muscle wasting,** ↓tone, ↓reflexes, ↓sensation. >**Sensory** - infective, metabolic, toxic, immune, nutritional Vit B. >**Motor** - Inflammatory Demyelinating Polyneuropathy (G-Barré).

3 **The neuro-muscular junction** *Proximal + eye muscle weakness* Myasthenia Gravis picture- Fatiguability: Ptosis - 'Battling to keep the eyes open, double vision'. Oropharnygeal - speaking, chewing, swallowing. Neostigmine response. AcCh receptor Abs±.

4 **The muscle** *Proximal myopathy-* Combing hair, stairs. **Myopathies** - metabolic **hypokalemia,** alcohol, endocrine, immune poly**myositis,** paraneoplastic. Consider hereditary muscular dystrophy Gowers+. **CK↑,** muscle biopsy, EMG.

Is this a generalized body weakness v. a true neurological weakness?

Stroke !ACUTE cerebrovascular incident

The key *Sudden onset* of 1-sided weakness, focal deficit.

Risks? Full stroke work-up.

| O/E: | Is it a stroke or TIA?

Anterior[1] v Posterior[2] circulation.

    Small vessel (lacunar[3]) **v large vessel** (cortex).

    Scan to distinguish **bleed v infarct**.

    Examine:

        heart - **ECG** ?rhythm. **CXR. Echo.**

        blood vessels ?Carotid bruit - bilateral dopplers

        risk factors.

Keep patient functional -Rehabilitate - speech - physio - OT.

Etiology -Make sure nothing missed to prevent further strokes.

| 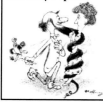 **Unusual causes of stroke Mr Spirochete 'the unsuitable suitor' and Lady Lupus** | Where no apparent pre-existing risk for stroke e.g. **young patient — consider an unusual** infective or immune **vasculitic cause or cardio-embolic source** such as MS, IE, or congenital heart lesion (e.g. ASD), atrial fibrillation; cerebral vessel malformation, or hypercoagulable state. To exclude occult vascular lesion or heart thrombus - bloods, Echo.

'I was struck by a stroke'. |

'The doctors made such a fuss - carotid study, scanned head;
In the end all I got was a disprin.'

Modify the modifiable - HT, aspirin,
statin, warfarin for AF.

A stroke strikes a patient. A gradual progressive onset of hemiparetic weakness is not in keeping with stroke -**fundo**scope - papilloedema. Brain Scan SOL? Non-vascular cause.

---

1   Weakness all same side - (Both the anterior and middle cerebral
     arteries are part of the anterior circulation - the carotids). Cortical.
2   Crossed signs - (cranial nn one side, motor/sensory other). Brainstem.
3   Deep white matter

11 THE ENDOCRINOLOGISTS

A recap to think 'glands'

General examination

1st impression
Too fat - DM Type 2, Cushing's
Too thin - hyperthyroidism, Addison's

Vitals
Endocrine HT

A more directed systemic examination

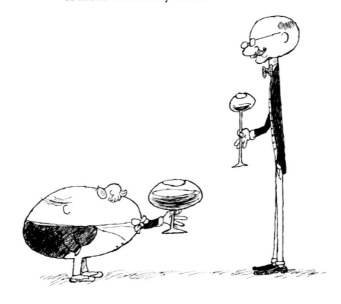

Obesity results from greater energy input than output.

Genes predispose to but don't cause obesity. The metabolic rate is regulated according to energy supply i.e. the lower the energy intake, the lower the metabolic rate and vice versa.

Body Mass Index

Excess adiposity makes examination difficult.

Strategy to reduce, maintain weight - diet, exercise.

Endocrine causes
Cushing's fat is centripetal - buffalo hump, striae.
  Hypothyroidism - weight gain is mild.
  PCOS - infertile, hairy female. Insulin resistance.

COMPLICATIONS OF OBESITY

Mechanical Overload

OA, varicose veins, small lung volumes, heavy snoring, sleep apnoea and pulmonary HT.

Metabolical overload

Address all CVS risks… A little too much - abdominal girth, BP, glucose, lipid, and **urate** are all part of this inter-related metabolic syndrome. Moderation in food and alcohol as well as adopting a less sedentary lifestyle - such as climbing stairs in lieu of using escalator. Physical activity sensitizes the body to insulin thereby reducing the risk of developing diabetes with all its attendant complications.

The patient has classical **features of insulin resistance –** which include a combination of telltale complementary signs- **acanthosis nigricans + skin tags** in the **neck and axillary folds, central obesity, HT, dyslipidemia, ± diabetes.** All these abnormal findings add up to make a collective diagnosis.

Diabetes mellitus

Is the no.1 endocrine disorder

Classical symptoms: polydipsia, **poly**uria, weakness.
> *'Insatiable thirst, blurred vision ... I shall visit my doctor.'*
U glu++ no ketones. Blood glucose↑ : **Type 2 DM.**

Lapsing into unconsciousness: **Type 1 DM** may present
dramatically with **DKA** - vomiting, dehydration, glycosuria and
ketonuria. Exclude a complicating infection.

> *'Adjusting to my new life...I shall have to comply with Rx.*
> *My HT seems to fit hand in glove with my diabetes'.*

Improve compliance. 'Fine-tune'- Tighten BP and glycemia
control to help delay the silent process of atherosclerosis.

Improve cardiometabolic profile

Adjusting the ups & downs ... normalise HbA₁c.
> **Match medication to mealtimes.** Consult dietician.
> **Bedtime snack** prevents **nocturnal hypoglycemia.**

> *'Nothing sweet passed my lips ... and so the years passed ...a very*
> *regular life.*
> *When my saliva gets dry - I know there's too much sugar in me.'*

'They discovered my Diabetes was ...' **due to a 2°cause:**
> *Endocrine:* gestation, steroid, acromegaly.
> *Pancreatic: Exclude calcifications* in a thin drinker and **Fe**
> *infiltration* in haemochromatosis – skin, hepar.

ALWAYS CHECK GLUCOSE
Dizziness, ↓ rousability ... Routine to check glucose!
Was u-dipstix checked?

In the line of duty...se-glucose

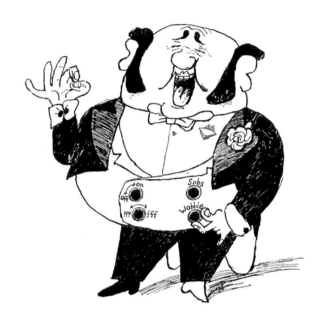

BEL CANTO

Patients referred to the Diabetes Clinic…

Monitor urine and blood glucose.

Examine phenotype (most patients are type 2).

Long-term vasculopathic complications.

ACUTE METABOLIC COMPLICATIONS

➤ *Hyperglycemia* Rx Interplay of oral medication and insulin.

➤ *Hypoglycemia* Shaky, sweaty spells - dextrose.

➤ *Ketoacidosis* Insufficient Insulin - a state of cell starvation.
Gluconeogenesis converts fatty acids to ketones. **Diagnosis of DKA made on hyperglycemia + ketonuria + glycosuria + acidosis (pH<7.3)**
Low CO_2 reflects HCO_3 level.

    FLUID + INSULIN: Start **normal saline** infusion to rehydrate + side-drip of fast-acting insulin.
    Monitor blood-glucose - when it falls below ~14 mmol, switch drip to 5% dextrose. **Interchange dextrose/saline** according to blood sugar levels.
    Continue insulin infusion until **no ketones** in **urine** - ensure patient has started eating to avoid starvation ketones. Change to maintenance Rx.

➤ *Hyperosmolar* Rx like DKA. Hydrate. Heparin-prone to clot!

WHO NEEDS TO INJECT SUBCUT. INSULIN?

▪ **Type 2: Supplement** if poorly controlled on maximal orals.
'I was on tablets for a long time. I became insulin dependent.'

[*In view of **persistently elevated glucose**, exclude infection. Check CXR. Consider PTB.*]

▪ **Type 1: Supplemental basal bolus regimen** ie long-acting nocte + short-acting at meals; or a more convenient mix b.d.

▪ **Pre-conception or pregnancy:** Switch to insulin.

▪ **Sliding scale:** Stress situation-sepsis, peri-op 5% dextrose.

CHRONIC VASCULOPATHIC COMPLICATIONS

➤ **Macroangiopathy:** atherosclerosis per se

Big infarcts are more **obvious.** Some patients present with **arterial occlusion: stroke, amputation, myocard infarct.**

'Heaviness in chest. Since then breathlessness.
I suffer cramps in the legs and sometimes in the heart.'

Silent cardiac ischaemia is attributed to autonomic neuropathy. Patient may have marked atherosclerosis such as ischaemic cardiomyopathy with relatively spared kidneys.
Oedema … cardiac or renal?

It may be wise to prescribe a **statin and low dose aspirin.**

➤ **Microangiopathy:** microinfarcts are more subtle

Equipped with **fundoscope, urine dipstix** and **monofilament** and **tuning fork** the meticulous diabetologist evaluates micro-circulation by **regularly screening eyes, kidneys and feet** for triad of **diabetic retinopathy, nephropathy, neuropathy.** Yearly **birthday eye check-up** may **prevent** blindness from exudative or proliferative **retinal changes** and early cataracts.

Have you checked feet and shins to identify DM foot at risk?

Inspectio: Underperfused **atrophic** and shiny skin = **dermopathy.**

Palpatio: Absent or feeble **foot pulses = peripheral vasculopathy.**

Percussio: Monofilament tests **sensation = small fibre neuropathy.**

Auscultatio: Tuning fork tests loss of **vibration** sense = **neuropathy.**

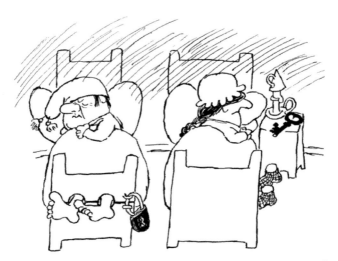

Nocturnal problems 'Feet are burning especially at night'

Neuro-vascular compromise: Diabetic neuropathy. PVD.

'My wife is an angel - she files my thickened toenails as skillfully as a podiatrist.' Keep feet dry - tinea pedis.

Sensory loss predisposes feet to callus, insensate injury, septic ulceration and delayed healing. Carbamazepine and amitriptyline alleviate the burning neuropathic pain.

'My wife complains' - **Rx erectile dysfunction accordingly.**

Cushing's Syndrome

Many who look Cushingoid have metabolic syndrome obesity - the **differential diagnosis.**

> **Exogenous** steroid is the **commonest cause.**
> **Endogenous** causes are uncommon:
> > - **adrenal cortex:** bilateral hyperplasia, adenoma, Ca.
> > - **pituitary:** micro or macroadenoma.

Corticosteroids exert **glucocorticoid, mineralocorticoid and weak androgenic** effects.

Glucocorticoids, being catabolic in action, promote *gluconeogenesis* as well as glycogenolysis. Protein substrate is also mobilized from skin, muscle and bone in order to raise blood glucose. This steroid-induced diabetogenic effect leads to poor wound healing.

> Sodium and water retention may cause steroid-induced HT.
> Androgenic effect stimulates the bone marrow cells.

Truncal obesity is striking. Rapid centripetal weight gain deposits fat in face, neck, between shoulder blades 'buffalo hump', abdomen (pendulous, wide red striae may develop in the same distribution).

Special Investigations:

Biochemical picture confirms **hypercortisolism.**

> Both serum cortisol and 24-hour urine cortisol↑.
> Serum ACTH is increased in pituitary Cushing's.
> **Radiology** ?Endogenous - Scan adrenals + pituitary.

As a general rule, prescribe the minimal effective cortisone dose to maintain desired therapeutic control. Taper/wean slowly.

Hirsutism

Androgenic over-expression

Cushing's e.g. virilizing congenital adrenal hyperplasia 2° enzyme↓, hypothyroidism, ovarian atrophy in menopause.

Insulin resistance PCOS - metformin restores ovulation.

Racial variation

$\boxed{\text{T}}$hyroid diseases Variable presentations

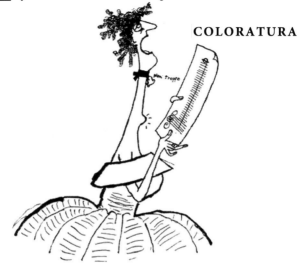

COLORATURA

Singing high metabolic notes

$\boxed{\text{H}}$yperthyroidism? $\boxed{\text{H}}$ypothyroidism?

$\boxed{\text{Y}}$ounger person with Graves' disease
Presents with symptoms and signs of thyroid hyperactivity -
palpitations, anxiety. $T_4\uparrow$, **TSH low**, thyroid antibodies.
Ask your patient to swallow liquid and observe a diffuse **goitre**
move up and become more prominent.
1 **Eye signs** - stare, proptosis, lid lag and retraction.
2 **Hand signs** - tremor, sweaty, onycholysis.
3 **The heart** bears the brunt of disease - **thyrocardiac disease**.
Older person tends to present in **AF, tachyarrythmia, HF.**
Apathetic hyperthyroidism is the paradoxical picture of loss of
energy in the absence of classical nervous thyrotoxic symptoms.
    Supportive Rx **beta-blocker and diuretic**.
Bridging antithyroid drug (Propylthiouracil / Carbimazole).
± Radio-ablation. Follow up thyroxine replacement.

Rate of metabolism *in every cell reflects thyroid hormone level.*

Older patient prone to hypothyroidism females > males
Hashimoto chronic thyroiditis: T$_4\downarrow$, **TSH high**, ± Abs.
   The not so obvious symptoms of hypoactive metabolism may
be missed for long. Tiredness, subtle changes of personality, lack
of memory, dry skin, weight gain, patient may appear a bit
neglected, macroglossia; coarseness of facial features and vocal
cords 2° to myxoedema. Easy to Rx. Replace thyroxine.
Monitor TSH + T$_4$ regularly - maintain euthyroid.

Investigations
Thyroid profile - **TSH** is the screening test.
T$_3$, T$_4$, and Abs to see whole picture.
   Imaging - Thyroid U/S. RAI-scan for thyrotoxicity.
   Cytology - of nodule - Ca commoner in younger person.

Different scenario - Surgeon's realm - Indications for
operation: Fear of Ca (FNA of nodule diagnostic / suspicious,
cervical nodes), pressure symptoms, unsightly endemic goitre or
hyperfunctioning nodule in multinodular goitre.

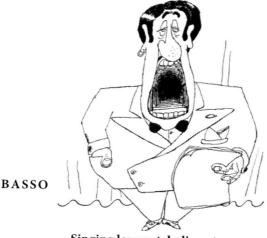

BASSO

Singing low metabolic notes

Pituitary presentations

In hormonal hierarchy the pituitary
is conductor of the endocrine system.

It's about pressure effects or hormone axis imbalance,
thus features of too little or too much.

Pressure symptoms - **headache** - ↑intracranial pressure.
      signs - **visual field defect** - loss of side vision.

Insufficient hypothalamic stimulating hormone/s
    (Pan) **hypopituitarism** ↓FSH, LH, TSH, ACTH.
    Too little hormone causes subtle signs and a real
disengagement with daily life. Pituitary hormone replacement
therapy reanimates the lacklustre - oestrogen/ testosterone,
thyroxine, cortisone.

Too much hormone
➤ Prolactinoma (most) - infertile, lactating - Rx bromocriptine
➤ Growth Hormone - acromegaly
➤ ACTH - Cushings - surgery if tumor circumscribed - RT.

To pick up a pituitary problem check:

- Pituitary hormone profile.
- Response to stimulation test(s). If no response→
- MRI pituitary to exclude macroadenoma.

Tall or short stature

Approach

Short + disproportionate = skeletal dysplasia
Short + proportionate:
➤ Constitutional (familial)
➤ Hormonal - excess or deficiency
➤ Chromosomal - Turner 45 X0; Klinefelter XXY
➤ Chronic disease or organ failure.

Look at hormones Growth H, thyroid H, cortisol.

Look at pituitary scan if indicated **and chromosomes.**

Male breast enlargement = gynaecomastia

Etiology: Too much estrogen /too little testosterone.
Drugs - digitalis, spironolactone, prostate Ca Rx.
Inherited - XXY Klinefelter-tall, hypogonadism.
Metabolic - alcoholic **cirrhosis**.
Malignancy - paraneoplastic - lung.
Mamma Ca - unilateral lump - biopsy
Testosterone↓ - pituitary tumour prolactinoma.
Obesity.
Physiological.

Normal 2° sexual development? Dysmorphic features?
Habitus, microgenitalia.
Hormones (think of pituitary axis to testis).
Scan pituitary to exclude adenoma.
Check visual fields.
Karyotype chromosomes.

Significant hypercalcemia

A high corrected calcium is easy to approach.
In the absence of a clear cause - check **PTH** level.

1 **Most are 2° to malignancy (Normal PTH)**
   Lytic mets - myeloma, breast. Rx Bisphosphonate.
   Paraneoplastic - PTH-like syndrome in bronchus Ca.
2 **1° Hyperparathyroidism ($\uparrow$ PTH)**
   Most parathyroid adenomas are asymptomatic and picked
   up incidentally. Kidney stones and HT are rare. 'Pepperpot'
   skull. Osteomalacia - bone pain or fracture. Post-op
   parathyroidectomy risk-hypocalcemic tetany.
3 **2° Hyperparathyroidism** (chronic renal failure).
4 **Iatrogenic** - calcium, vit D.

Insignificantly raised Calcium in **granulomatous diseases** -
TB, Sarcoid.

$\boxed{\text{A}}$ddison's disease [Adrenal insufficiency]

$\boxed{\text{D}}$**epletion of steroid, salt, sugar.** Chronically ill patient.
Picked up on **low BP, low Na$^+$, high K$^+$.** Confirm on low se-
cortisol. Hyperpigmented patient. Chronic auto-immune
condition or HIV-TB-related.

   Acute Addisonian crisis= **Shock picture** 2° to abrupt
withdrawal of long-term steroid as the hypothalamic-
hypophyseal-adrenal axis is suppressed. Stress, e.g. infection or
op precipitates dramatic GIT symptoms, dehydration.

   Cortisone - life saving. **Fluid**-dextrose/ saline drip.

$\boxed{\text{R}}$**eplace** Gluco ± mineralocorticoid in autoimmune case.

Other causes of a low Na$^+$ include:

1 **Pseudo**-drugs e.g. carbamezepine.
2 **Under-hydration** or **over-hydration**.
3 **SIADH** $\downarrow$Na, Cl, osmolarity:
      Paraneoplastic - small cell Ca lung.
      Chronic lung or meningeal TB.
4 **Salt-losing nephropathy.**

12 THE GERONTOLOGISTS

from the Greek geron = old man

Domain of mature medicine

Adjusting to the difficulties of old age
Multiple organ degeneration gradually acclimatizes
the ageing person to intermittent symptoms such as wheezing,
pedal oedema, joint pains and backache.

Is the condition recoverable?
'Treat the treatables, reverse the reversibles, correct the
correctables'.

Epitaph

He was a very cautious man,
Who never laughed or played.
He rarely smiled, he never dreamed
Nor kissed a pretty maid.

So, when at last he died, they say,
Insurance was denied
Because he'd never really lived
They claimed he never died.

(Composed by an English priest)

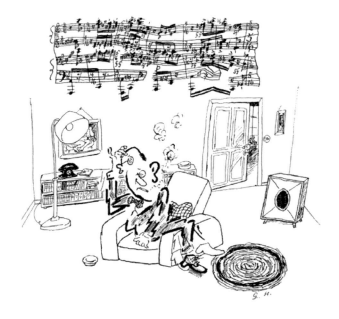

Why is he not talking to us?

A confusional state or **prolonged delirium** is a common presentation in the elderly. Encephalopathy is impaired brain function resulting from toxic, organic, infective, ischaemic or metabolic causes. Old people get very sick - they recover slowly - but they do recover.

Organ degeneration

Explains gradual decline of function. One small shift in tissue perfusion and oxygenation may tip a fragile haemodynamic scale to effect an earlier and more profound disturbance than in youth. For example, a **urinary tract infection** may **induce vomiting, dehydration and pre-renal failure**, all of which contribute to be optimal and appropriate to physiological function.

Mild anemia may promote **angina** - and **iatrogenic fluid** can **overload** a compromised heart into **pulmonary oedema**.

It is more dramatic in the surgical setting where a patient is exposed to insults of bleeding and anaesthesia. Single organ failure, e.g. acute renal failure, rapidly snowballs to involve other organ systems.

Loss of organ function[1]

Cognition ... sight ... dentition ... free movement.

Decreased organ reserves[2]

Optimize Rx, finding the balance, as you would in a younger patient, with consideration for a slower pharmacokinetic profile, hence the elderly's **susceptibility to drug toxicity**.

Post-stroke rehabilitation minimizes loss of function. Where possible, **mobilise with physio** to get patient back on his feet.

---

1   'He is deaf. He can't walk far, nor see far. Despite missing teeth he enjoys his food. He is forgetful. He gives a sign when he wants something. He responds well to attention and comes alive with love. He really holds onto life'.

2   'My heart reacts too slowly. The breath runs out. If I sit my breath is fine. If I walk quickly, then my lungs are too slow for the steps I take. If I sit I'm just as healthy as you.

   You must not hurry me, then it is too quick: the earth turns quicker than me; the earth turns once in 24 hours.

   I won a running trophy at school. I remember things I did when I was 6, but not what I did last week. I've become slower - But I'm simpler, I speak more directly, I do not use compensated words.'

DELICATE BALANCE

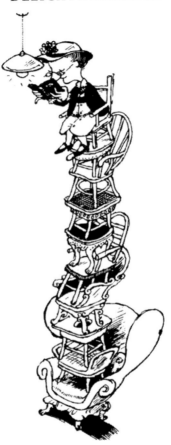

Old people have little reserves to compensate and thus decompensate 'at the drop of a hat'. A compromised system merely needs another incident to exceed its functional limit.

When more than one organ *plays out of tune*

A **system run-down** appreciates the **many degenerative problems and diseases** that an ageing person has to accept:

➤ **brain***
➤ **ears, eyes, teeth**
➤ **endocrine** - DM, thyroid
➤ **lungs**
➤ **heart**
➤ **GIT**
➤ **prostate and other neoplasms**
➤ **GU**
➤ **extremities** - arthritis, falls, fracture, circulation
   et cetera...

'CREEPING INFIRMITIES OF OLD AGE'

Symptomatic Rx

Some drugs work especially well. **Furosemide** is a potent **loop diuretic** -resulting in a dramatic response if the patient is in **heart failure**. After that, s/he feels s/he can live; If precipitant is an infection, an antibiotic helps complete the recovery.

*Decreased brain reserve
   1°Degenerative dementia - Alzheimer, vascular, P'plus.
   2°Acquired - B₁₂, thyroid↕, brain - trauma, tumour, infection.

A demented patient can deteriorate due to 2° causes e.g. **pneumonia** is the **'old man's friend'** and **UTI** the **'old lady's'**.

Slowing down '*I am in the wars ... I'm on the mend, but still a bit washed out. I'm house-bound. To add to my woes the knee gout has come back again. I'm a bit knocked for six, never mind, it's a germ. I'm out of steam. I'm out of action altogether.*'

In retrospect, What Will I Remember?

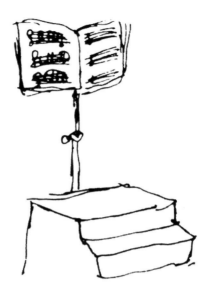

I will not jump to conclusions.
Check patient history.
General overview.
Systematic examination.
I will reserve my judgement till the end.
Stand back and pause to consider the options.
Re-spect = Re-check.
Consider a more extensive diff diagnosis - think of all the possible causes at the bedside.
Review all signs. Cover the basis of a sign.
Problem statement and summary.

Promotio
Cacophony is subsiding.
I am now experiencing **harmony***.*

Signs are becoming more evident.
A real breakthrough: their likely etiologies are starting to appear.

Reassurance comes from the continued practicum of our appropriate response to these signals of disease.

I always **aim to reach the root of the problem** in the shortest possible time. That is why the discipline of conducting the **three movements** of a diagnostic process is the key to success!

Strong in signs, strong in diagnosis.

With every problem we are invited to embark on our own *via diagnostica***, a veritable journey of growing awareness and observation.**

Each presentation is unclassically classical.
Appreciate the key notes of each disease and the sounds of a diagnosis will become music to your ears!

List of abbreviations

Abs	antibodies
ABG	arterial blood gas
ACE	angiotensin converting enzyme
AcCh	acetylcholine
ACTH	adrenocorticotropic hormone
ADA	adenosine deaminase
AF	atrial fibrillation
AFB	acid fast bacilli
AFP	alpha fetoprotein
AGN	acute glomerulonephritis
AI	aortic incompetence
ALL	acute lymphatic leukaemia
ALP	alkaline phosphatase
ANCA	anti-neutrophil cytoplasmic antibody
ANF	anti-nuclear factor
ARF	acute renal failure
AS	aortic valve stenosis
ASD	atrial septal defect
ASO	anti-streptolysin O
ATN	acute tubular necrosis
BM	bone marrow
BP	blood pressure
BR	bilirubin
BVF	biventricular failure
Ca	carcinoma
CAP	community acquired pneumonia
CCF	congestive cardiac failure
CEA	carcinoembryonic antigen
CK	creatine kinase
CLL	chronic lymphatic leukaemia
CML	chronic myeloid leukaemia
CMO	cardiomyopathy
CMV	cytomegalovirus
COPD	chronic obstructive pulmonary disease
CPR	cardio-pulmonary resuscitation
CRF	chronic renal failure
CRP	C-Reactive protein
CSF	cerebrospinal fluid
CT	computed tomography
CVI	cerebrovascular incident
CVS	cardiovascular system

CXR	chest X-ray
DIC	disseminated intravascular coagulation
DKA	diabetic ketoacidosis
DIP	distal interphalangeal
DM	diabetes mellitus
DTs	delirium tremens
DVT	deep venous thrombosis
EBV	Epstein Barr virus
ECG	electrocardiogram
EEG	electroencephalogram
EMG	electromyogram
ENT	ear, nose & throat
ESR	erythrocyte sedimentation rate
FBC	full blood count
FEV_1	forced expiratory volume in 1 second
FVC	forced vital capacity
FNA	fine needle aspirate
GCS	Glasgow coma scale
GE	gastro-enteritis
GERD	gastro-oesophageal reflux disease
GGT	gamma-glutamyl transferase
GI	gastro-intestinal
GIT	gastro-intestinal tract
GN	glomerulonephritis
Gram	gram +/- organisms
Hb	haemoglobin
HD	heart disease
HF	heart failure
HIV	human immunodeficiency virus
HOCM	hypertrophic obstructive cardiomyopathy
HSM	hepatosplenomegaly
HT	hypertension
IBD	inflammatory bowel disease
ICS	intercostal space
IDDM	insulin dependent diabetes mellitus
IE	infective endocarditis
Ig	immunoglobulin
ILD	interstitial lung disease
ITP	idiopathic thrombocytopenic purpura
i.v.	intravenous
JVP	jugular venous pressure
LA	left atrium
LDH	lactate dehydrogenase
LFT	liver function tests

LHF	left heart failure
LICS	left intercostal space
LMN	lower motor neuron
LN	lymphnode
LP	lumbar puncture
LUL	left upper lobe
LV	left ventricle
LVF	left ventricular failure
LVH	left ventricular hypertrophy
MCL	mid-clavicular line
MCP	metacarpophalangeal
MCS	microscopy, culture & sensitivity
MCV	mean corpuscular volume
MI	myocardial infarction
MR	mitral regurgitation
MRI	magnetic resonance imaging
MS	mitral valve stenosis
MV	mitral valve
MVP	mitral valve prolapse
NSAIDs	non-steroidal anti-inflammatory drugs
OA	osteoarthritis
OD	overdose
O/E	on examination
OT	occupational therapy
PA	pulmonary artery
PCOS	polycystic ovarian syndrome
PDA	patent ductus arteriosus
PEF	peak expiratory flow
PHT	pulmonary hypertension
PIP	proximal interphalangeal
PN	pyelonephritis
PND	paroxsymal nocturnal dyspnoea
PS	pulmonary stenosis
PSA	prostate specific antigen
PTB	pulmonary tuberculosis
PTED	pulmonary thromboembolic disease
PTH	parathyroid hormone
PUO	pyrexia of unknown origin
PVD	peripheral vascular disease
RA	rheumatoid arthritis
RAI	radio-active iodine
RBC	red blood cell
RES	reticulo endothelial system
RF	rheumatic fever

RHF	right heart failure
RIC	right intercostal space
RML	right middle lobe
RR	Respiratory Rate
RT	radiotherapy
RV	right ventricle
RVF	right ventricular failure
RVH	right ventricular hypertrophy
Rx	treatment
SA	sino-atrial node
SBP	spontaneous bacterial peritonitis
SBE	subacute bacterial endocarditis
SIADH	syndrome of inappropriate anti-diuretic hormone
SLE	systemic lupus erythematosus
SOL	space-occupying lesion
STD	sexually transmitted disease
SVCO	superior vena cava obstruction
T°	temperature
T4	forth thoracic vertebra
TB	tuberculosis
TFT	thyroid function tests
TI	tricuspid incompetence
TIA	transient ischaemic attack
TOF	tetralogy of Fallot
TSH	thyroid stimulating hormone
TV	tricuspid valve
U+E	urea, electrolytes, & creatinine
UMN	upper motor neuron
U/S	ultrasound
UT	urinary tract
UTI	urinary tract infection
VEs	ventricular ectopics
VSD	ventricular septal defect
WCC	white cell count
WR	Wasserman reaction /syphilis serology